VACCINE ROUNDUP

Should I have one of the COVID-19 coronavirus vaccinations?

Questioning the narrative: an exercise in critical thought

Ian Usher

Vaccine Roundup

Should I have one of the COVID-19 coronavirus vaccinations?

Questioning the narrative: an exercise in critical thought

Ian Usher

VaccineRoundup.com

CONTENTS

INTRODUCTION

"Pandemic is not a word to use lightly or carelessly. It is a word that, if misused, can cause unreasonable fear, or unjustified acceptance that the fight is over, leading to unnecessary suffering and death."

Dr. Tedros Adhanom Ghebreyesus

WHO Director-General

11th March 2020

Please come in for your appointment

The phone rings and you pick up. It's one of the nurses from your local health facility. You are invited to come along tomorrow to one of the new inoculation centres that have been set up to fast-track vaccinations against the SARS-CoV-2 virus.

In the background over the phoneline you can hear the hum of many other voices, and you realise that there are other nurses making similar calls to other people on the health clinic's database.

The big push is on to protect the world against COVID-19, the disease caused by the virus, and you can play your small role by lining up to have your shot.

It's decision time. Are you ready to take part in the biggest vaccine roll-out the world has ever seen?

If I ruled the world...

When you were growing up, did you ever play the game, "If I ruled the world..."?

It may have been called "King for a day", or it may have simply been posed as a question: "What would you do if you were in charge?"

As a kid, perhaps you dreamed of a never-ending supply of chocolate, or a big castle filled with your favourite toys? Did you want to ban school, or have a stable filled with ponies?

As an adult offered the role of global leadership, you might be a little less self-centred, and perhaps consider how you could make the world a better place.

Maybe you've even played your own version of this game recently?

The challenges we currently face as a planet – there are plenty of them – may have prompted you to wonder how you might handle these issues, should you be given the power to do so.

One of our current global dilemmas – the coronavirus crisis – may have also prompted you to question the sudden shifts happening around us, as our governments subject us to all sorts of policy changes in order to tackle a virus that has swept around the world.

It is almost impossible to side-step the consequences of the restrictions that have been enforced to varying degrees in different parts of the world, and it would seem quite clear that we aren't going to be returning to the "old normal" of January 2020 any time soon.

You'll no doubt be familiar with common new phraseology, such as, "unprecedented times" and "the new normal". Perhaps you've also heard the terms "vaccine hesitancy", "vaccine denier" or "anti-vaxxer".

Over the course of 2020 there was much discussion of a potential vaccine for COVID-19, the disease caused by the SARS-CoV-2 virus. In the early days of the pandemic a commonly touted timeline for vaccine production was "12 to 18 months".

It was often suggested that this timeline was a very optimistic best-case scenario, as no vaccine had ever been produced in such a short time. Most vaccines take years to create, and then more years to test for both safety and efficacy.

But here we are, in early February 2021, less than a year since most of us had any idea that our lives were about to change so dramatically, and a vaccine has already been administered to millions of people around the world.

So, right now we're all facing a choice. Do we get in line to have a COVID-19 vaccine, or do we join the ranks of "vaccine deniers" and refuse to be inoculated?

The goal of this book is to help you to make that decision.

So, who am I, and what qualifies me to write on this topic?

My name is Ian Usher, and I was born in 1963 in the UK. One of my major passions is travel, and I've visited over 60 countries, and lived in several, including Australia, Canada, Panama and Mexico.

As I write this I am living in France, since being locked down here for a month in November of 2020. I have decided to stay on here for a while.

So much of what follows in this book will have a bit of a UK / European slant, but that won't really matter, as the topics we'll look at together are generally global in nature.

Let's begin with full disclosure:

1. **I have no medical qualifications whatsoever**... I imagine most people reading this don't either. But I am fortunate enough to be in a position where I only have to work on a part-time basis. This gives me the time to research, to consider, to question.

2. **I don't have any answers for you.** The choices you make for yourself are yours and yours alone. Your circumstances are undoubtedly different to mine, and will therefore shape your decision-making process in a very personal manner.

3. **I can't give you any "facts" and I don't know "the truth".** All I can offer are some thoughts, some questions, and my own opinions based on information available to all of us, albeit it at times requiring some deep searching to unearth it. In fact, I'll go as far as to suggest that you should have a healthy degree of scepticism for anything presented to you as "the truth" or "the facts". As we'll see later, truth can be a very slippery concept these days.

4. **I am not an anti-vaxxer.** I have had vaccinations in the past, first of all as a child growing up in the UK, then later as a young adult I had a couple of booster shots. The last vaccine I was given was in 2010 when, to be allowed to enter Brazil, I had to have a Yellow Fever vaccination. The choice was either accept the jab and get the certificate, or forget "bucket list" plans to go to Carnival in Rio.

5. **I have no political leanings.** I am generally uninterested in politics, and firmly agree with George Carlin, who is quoted later in the book, when he says, "Forget the politicians, they're irrelevant." Unfortunately, in the situation we currently find ourselves in, we do have to pay attention to their decisions, as they are having significant impact on our daily lives. However, for example,when I mention Donald Trump or Boris Johnson, I don't intend to imply either support of or criticism for any particular side of the political divide.

6. **Finally, It's quite possible that this book will earn me (and possibly you too for reading it) the label of "conspiracy theorist".** We'll look at the subject of labelling later in the book, but again, in the spirit of full disclosure, my personal decision (for now) is not to be vaccinated.

So with those points clarified, what can you hope to gain from reading this book?

My goal is simple... to give you a few topics to consider and a few ideas to examine, before you jump in and get vaccinated.

I want to help you to be able to think carefully and clearly about what is happening around you. I hope to inspire you to question the current narrative around our global dilemma.

And I would like to give you some critical thinking tools to help you examine things from all sides, before you make your final decision.

So let's get started.

We'll begin with an overview of the stories we are told...

PART 1: THE STORIES WE'RE TOLD

"If you tell a big enough lie and tell it frequently enough, it will be believed."

Adolf Hitler

Pandemic!

You know the story as well as I do, I imagine. 2020 was a challenging year for all of us.

In January, news of a new coronavirus outbreak started coming out of China, and the World Health Organization (WHO) was monitoring the situation.

In Wuhan, centre of the outbreak, people were asked to stay at home, businesses were closed, and movement was severely restricted. It wasn't until February that most people outside China started to become aware of what was going on.

The world looked on in shock and amazement as stories of people being locked in and doors welded shut started to surface. Eerie videos of silent, empty streets, and distressing footage of people dying in over-filled hospital corridors stunned the world.

Slowly the realisation dawned that this virus had a significant potential to spread to other countries, and the word "pandemic" became a part of our vocabulary.

For a while it looked like Japan, Singapore and South Korea were going to be the hardest hit. Cruise ships became a focal point as the disease spread and people were quarantined aboard the Diamond Princess.

Europe and the USA became the next hotspots, and Italy, particularly the northern part of the country, was hit hard. Numbers started rising in France, Spain and the UK too.

The disease progression started with a dry cough and a fever, and in some cases led to severe breathing difficulties. This often resulted in hospitalisation and the need for an Intensive Care Unit (ICU) bed. The most severe cases needed assistance to breathe via a respirator, and many of these cases eventually resulted in death.

Borders closed and many countries began restricting flights in and out of their territory. The world started closing down, which merely exacerbated the logistical issue which had begun when China closed most of its manufacturing capacity in January.

Advice from the WHO and governments tended to be contradictory at times, and disagreement raged over whether masks should be worn by people at all times when out and about. Most western countries' health organisations advised against mask use, as did the WHO.

The WHO finally designated the outbreak as a "pandemic" on 11th March, by which point the virus had spread to 110 countries around the world.[1]

In many of these countries it quickly became apparent that there was the potential for the health system to become overwhelmed.

As numbers of cases climbed, hospital wards filled and supply problems meant that there wasn't enough Personal Protective Equipment (PPE) for hospital staff. If numbers kept climbing, potentially hospitals weren't going to have enough ICU beds, enough respirators, or enough staff to look after the sudden influx of patients in desperate need of help.

Rising case numbers were followed days or weeks later by an increase in deaths, and panic mounted around the globe. Further measures were obviously going to be needed to slow the spread of the virus and "flatten the curve", giving hospitals a fighting chance to deal this unfolding situation.

China seemed to have controlled their outbreak by severely restricting the movements of their citizens, and a new term became common. "Lockdowns" had arrived.

In the UK in late March the whole country was locked down, and all movement was restricted to only the most essential services. It was initially suggested that the lockdown would last two weeks. It didn't end until early July, some 15 weeks later.

Other countries employed similar tactics to varying degrees, with varying levels of success.

Throughout the lockdowns the state of the economy was a major concern for every country in the world too. Governments were caught between a rock and a hard place. Locking down the population meant closing down most businesses, with potentially disastrous consequences. Allowing freedom of movement would permit the virus to spread more quickly, and potentially overwhelm health systems.

Different countries came up with different solutions to try to stave off the worst of the economic fallout. In the UK a furlough scheme was introduced, whereby people unable to go to work could apply to receive 80% of their regular salary, up to a maximum monthly payout of £2,000, from the government.[2]

---

1 https://time.com/5791661/who-coronavirus-pandemic-declaration/

2 https://www.gov.uk/coronavirus/business-support

In the USA the government sent out occasional "stimulus checks" to most citizens, and introduced the Paycheck Protection Program, which provides loans to help businesses keep their workforce employed during the crisis.[3] It has been suggested that many of these loans will never need to be paid back, so in effect this is a very similar program to the UK's furlough scheme.

Over the latter part of the summer, as case numbers dropped, restrictions eased, travel resumed, to a degree at least, and some semblance of getting back to regular routines made life feel more normal once more.

With supply chains now able to keep up with demand for masks for personal use, some governments made U-turns on their earlier advisories, and masks now started to become obligatory in most indoor spaces, and hand sanitizer could be found at the entrance of most stores. Customer numbers were still limited, and "social distancing" remained a high priority.

There was much talk of "the new normal", and of a potential "second wave" of the disease.

There was also lots of talk of a vaccine, and the oft-touted, optimistic timeline of vaccine development of a minimum of 12 to 18 months. But as autumn approached the sense of foreboding grew.

In October in many countries, the "second wave" was fast approaching, as numbers of infections began to climb, although initially the death count stubbornly refused to follow suit. Of course, by this time we'd learned much more about the disease, and had more efficient treatment regimes, so perhaps this was the reason. Most countries were also doing a lot more testing.

The only way out of this dilemma would appear to be a miraculously early development of a vaccine. According to the WHO and most western government guidelines, as of October 2020, there wasn't any real effective way to protect people from the virus.

In the UK people who tested positive were simply told to go home, self-isolate, and return for further medical assistance if symptoms developed to a serious degree. There was a suggestion that small doses of Vitamin D might be helpful in the protection of older members of the community.

As November approached the lockdowns began in earnest again in France, UK, Spain, Italy and various parts of the USA. Fear and despair began to

---

[3] https://www.sba.gov/funding-programs/loans/coronavirus-relief-options/paycheck-protection-program

mount as businesses closed and our horizons narrowed once more to the little world around us.

However, a surprise announcement on 9th November offered a huge ray of hope. Pharma giant Pfizer, in partnership with BioNTech, had developed a vaccine which, in Stage 3 trials, had proven to be 90% effective.

Within days there was another announcement, this time from pharma company Moderna. They too had developed a vaccine with a similar success rate. And yet another, in the UK, from a partnership between University of Oxford and pharma company AstraZeneca.

There were words of caution. It would take time to produce enough doses of the vaccines for everyone in the world. The Pfizer vaccine in particular had logistical challenges, in that it had to be stored at extremely low temperatures.

Within weeks Emergency Use Authorization (EUA) applications were received by the U.S. Food and Drug Administration (FDA). Governments around the world were lining up to buy as many shots of the new vaccines as possible.

According to Wikipedia, "by December, more than 10 billion vaccine doses had been preordered by countries, with about half of the doses purchased by high-income countries comprising only 14% of the world's population."[4]

Under the leadership of Boris Johnson, the UK was among the first countries to get hold of the vaccine, and with much fanfare and press coverage, on Tuesday December 8th 2020, Margaret Keenan from Northern Ireland, a 90-year-old grandmother, became the first person in the world to receive the Pfizer vaccine (outside of vaccine trials).[5]

There was much prevarication about "opening up" for Christmas, leaders torn between the need to slow the spread of the virus, while still allowing people the ability to share some time with loved ones.

I imagine your Christmas in 2020 was very different from the one you enjoyed in 2019.

Now in early 2021, with numbers of cases still high, hospitals apparently approaching capacity, and the death tally still mounting, it seems the race is on to get everyone vaccinated in the shortest possible timeframe.

---

[4] https://en.wikipedia.org/wiki/COVID-19_vaccine

[5] https://www.reuters.com/article/uk-health-coronavirus-britain-idUSKBN28I0OQ

News of "new variants" of the virus keep surfacing, each one potentially more transmissive or more deadly than previous versions. There is much discussion about whether the current vaccines will be effective against these new strains. Perhaps the vaccines will need to be "tweaked" to have a broader range of effectiveness. Perhaps we will need booster shots to add immunisation for new variants of the virus as they emerge.

The breathless state of government panic and media hype seems to be ever-on-going, with European countries now back-stabbing each other over vaccine supplies. Vaccine companies are suggesting they may not be able to provide supplies at the rate they initially promised and contracted for.

The UK government has decided that they will administer as many first shots of a vaccine as possible, and against the manufacturer's initial guidelines, will delay giving the second shot from the advised 3 weeks out to 12 weeks.

Much of Europe is under one form or another of lockdown, curfew, or restriction of movement. Most countries now have mask mandates, usually when in enclosed spaces, many "non-essential" businesses remain closed, and movement between regions is discouraged.

In most cases travel to another country, particularly if flying, requires a negative result from a Polymerase Chain Reaction[6] (PCR) test within 72 hours before the flight. France has closed its borders for both incoming and outgoing travel to countries outside the EU.

Since 15th February 2021 the UK government has implemented the use of "quarantine hotels", where incoming travellers have to pay for 10 days of isolation before being allowed to join the general populace. At first it wasn't clear whether this would be for everyone, regardless of where they were arriving from. However, with a little more clarity provided at the last minute, this strategy is currently used for inbound travellers from countries on the UK Government's so-called "red list"[7] where new variant strains of the virus are appearing.

The story we are told every day is that only a successful worldwide roll-out of vaccinations can allow us to make any steps back towards some sort of normality.

---

[6] https://www.genome.gov/about-genomics/fact-sheets/Polymerase-Chain-Reaction-Fact-Sheet

[7] https://www.gov.uk/guidance/transport-measures-to-protect-the-uk-from-variant-strains-of-covid-19#travel-bans-to-the-uk---banned-countries

The narrative

A term that is often heard in relation to the pandemic and the roll-out of vaccines is "the narrative".

I used this term in the introduction, stating, "I hope to inspire you to question the current narrative around our global dilemma." Throughout this book I'll often refer to the story we're told about what is going on around us as "the narrative".

But what exactly does this term mean?

From the Cambridge Dictionary one definition of a narrative is: "a particular way of explaining or understanding events"

The in-context example from the Cambridge Dictionary of using the term in this way is: "There was pressure on academics to construct narratives of the period that were positive."[8]

In other words, the narrative is the same as "spin" – telling a story in a way that puts certain events in a context that suits a particular goal or desired outcome.

Those who control the narrative, who feed us the stories that we are asked to believe, have incredible power to shape our thoughts, beliefs, and ultimately the choices we make and the actions we take.

We'll look later at the issue of censorship, and how it would appear that many credible sources who put forward ideas that "don't fit the narrative" are being ignored, or even worse, silenced.

Why would a society that values free speech – freedom of expression is proudly touted as the First Amendment of the U.S. Constitution – want to silence those who have ideas, suggestions, or evidence that contradict the main story we are being told?

It would seem self-evident that if someone is telling the truth they don't need a "narrative". If they are telling the truth, conflicting ideas and opinions would not need to be censored or smothered, as eventually the truth would be obvious to all.

We'll delve further into different alternatives to the main narrative in Part 4.

---

[8] https://dictionary.cambridge.org/dictionary/english/narrative

The economy

Before the coronavirus crisis hit us, how many times did we hear Donald Trump proudly declare that the USA was enjoying a period of strong growth, that this was "the greatest economy in the world", and that all was going great under his leadership?

Using the stock market as the main measure of the economy certainly offered a rosy picture, as there were often reports of different market indices hitting new all-time highs..

However, many economists in the background were sounding alarms. The bailouts after the 2007-2008 financial crisis had merely papered over the cracks in the crumbling system, many claimed. With massive injections of monetary stimulus, euphemistically referred to as Quantitative Easing, the stock market had benefitted from the newly created currency sloshing around in the system, and had rallied over the following decade, giving Trump his "greatest economy" credentials.

But easy credit and interest rates held at artificially low rates helped huge levels of debt to build in auto (car) loans, student loans and the bond market, much as it had done in the housing sector a decade earlier. Again, some economists predicted that the crash we experienced in 2008 was not over, and that there was much worse to come. The bubble that had popped in 2008 in the housing market had been re-inflated to much greater proportions, this time in multiple sectors of the economy.

At the end of 2019, to many economists, certain sectors of the market were looking very precarious. Then as we entered 2020 our world shifted around us, and the focus of our collective concerns shifted to a new crisis.

So, how does the economy look now, a year later as we head into 2021, and we look to vaccines as the magic bullet to get us out of the crisis and back to a "new normal"?

I don't think I need to defend myself against potential accusations of being a "conspiracy theorist" if I say that the outlook for the economy in many countries looks dire. Many economists are now predicting a "lost decade" as we look to the future, and this almost seems inevitable.

So many businesses have closed their doors, having been hit hard by lockdowns. The bigger players in the travel industry, such as airlines, cruises, holiday and theme parks, as well as many other holiday operators have suffered devastating losses.

Closer to home, restaurants, bars and high street shops of all types have been closed, and income has fallen off a cliff.

All of these businesses rely on suppliers, manufacturers and other service providers, all of which will be suffering terrible hardship too.

In the UK a government furlough scheme[9], which pays a substantial portion of workers' wages if they have been unable to work as normal, was implemented at the start of the first lockdown, in March 2020.

The furlough scheme was originally due to expire in June, and was extended to the end of the year. As lockdowns returned in November a further extension to the end of March 2021 was announced. This was an obvious indication that the government was expecting a bad winter.

In December another extension was added, taking the furlough out to the end of April 2021.

This furlough is currently hiding the full damage that has been done to the economy, as many companies are hanging on desperately while the government covers the wages of their staff. There must be hundreds of thousands of people currently "employed" and being salaried by the government.

When the furlough is eventually wound down there are going to be countless businesses unable to return to paying their staff, as their emergency funds, if they had any, will be severely depleted. This will likely translate into millions of people who suddenly find themselves unemployed.

Any of these who have large debts, such as a mortgage on their home, will soon fall into arrears, unless they have significant savings put away. Houses will be put up for sale, but with a glut of properties all hitting the market at the same time, there will be a huge downward pressure on prices. A few months later the repossessions will begin, just as they did in 2008.

Once again, caught between a rock and a hard place, the government faces another lose-lose choice. They can either let the inevitable tsunami of unemployment happen, and hope to deal with the fallout afterwards, or they can keep paying furlough payments, or perhaps even transition to the much-talked-about Universal Basic Income (UBI).

The question this raises is an obvious one. Where will all the money come from?

The answer doesn't offer much hope. It will be printed up, created out of thin air... or rather than actually printing anything, a few strokes on a keyboard, and "Hey Presto!", new money is available to distribute as needed.

---

[9] https://www.gov.uk/coronavirus/business-support

The obvious downside to this solution is a dilution of the currency supply as more currency units are created, with the predictable consequences of price inflation, as more cash circulates, bidding for the same, or perhaps shrinking supply of goods.

Most of the western world will fare no better than the UK, some perhaps much worse. The European Central Bank (ECB) has fired up the printing presses, as has the Federal Reserve in the USA.

What could possibly go wrong?

Fake news

Donald Trump was always quick to use the term "fake news" when the story being told didn't gel with his version of reality. He wasn't always correct in his use of the term, as he often used it to label articles that showed him in a bad light.

The idea behind any "fake news" claim is that the media is used as a tool to manipulate what people believe, and thus influence their choices or behaviour. Here's a useful definition[10]:

> The term fake news means "news articles that are intentionally and verifiably false" designed to manipulate people's perceptions of real facts, events, and statements.

We'll look more closely at the media later on, when we discuss "the people we trust" and "the assumptions we make".

For now though, it's important to bear in mind that all of "the stories we're told" are related to us via one form of media or another.

Maybe you get your news from the TV. There are many 24-hours-a-day news services. Some of these channels will have known political leanings in one direction or another.

Perhaps you source your information online, from one of the major news websites, via news aggregators such as Microsoft News or Google News.

Or maybe you have a favourite newspaper, either national or local, which you can read either online, or in the more traditional paper format.

Social networks such as Facebook and Twitter also offer news articles and information.

And of course YouTube, owned by Google, offers a wealth of news in video format from a huge range of sources. You can access information from large media news outlets, small independents, and individual citizen journalists.

How do we know that the stories they tell us are true, or whether what we are watching or reading is "fake news"? Are our perceptions of real facts, events and statements being manipulated by articles designed to make us think and act in certain ways?

In the modern world, swamped under a deluge of possible sources of varying credibility, is it ever really possible for any of us to know what the truth actually is?

---

[10] https://www.cits.ucsb.edu/fake-news/what-is-fake-news

PART 2:
THE PEOPLE WE TRUST

“For there to be betrayal, there would have to have been trust first.”

Suzanne Collins

The Hunger Games

Who rules the world?

We all live within the rules and boundaries of one or other of the world's (approximately) 200 countries. In the westernized world, most countries have similar systems of government, in which we have two or more political parties. These parties have a chosen leader, and through a system of national elections, a winning party is selected, and a President, Prime Minister, or Premier is chosen for the country.

Are these the people who rule the world?

They usually hold office for a set number of years, and then have to face the challenge of securing re-election if they want further time in office. They don't have the power to hold office for as long as they might like, as a dictator under a different system of governance might be able to do.

Their major function is the day-to-day management of the country, as well as consideration of longer term strategies for future development, in much the same way a CEO oversees the running of a large company.

They have a degree of decision-making power at a national level, and as we've seen over the past year or so, their policies can have a huge impact on the daily lives of their citizens... you and me.

But I think we're safe to say that on a global level, for the leaders of most countries, their power and reach is limited. Obviously some countries are bigger players on the international stage than others, involving themselves in the affairs of other nations to a greater degree than smaller powers.

So who makes the decisions and sets the policies at a higher level than national governments?

Let's take a little peek down the entrance of the rabbit hole...

There is a suggestion of an unknown number of international bodies, organisations, think tanks, groups, and private clubs who gather, sometimes in the open, sometimes in clandestine secrecy, to consider global issues.

Well known international organisations who make decisions and set policies which affect the lives of more people than the citizens of just one country include, but is not limited to, the UN (United Nations)[11], the IMF (International Monetary Fund)[12], the EU (European Union)[13], OPEC

---

11 https://www.un.org/en/

12 https://www.imf.org/en/Home

13 https://europa.eu/european-union/index_en

(Organization of the Petroleum Exporting Countries)[14] and the WEF (World Economic Forum)[15].

Beyond these international bodies, there are business entities which have huge international influence. The food industry, Big Pharma, social media giants, and huge traditional media enterprises all affect the lives of millions, if not billions of people around the globe. We'll look in a bit more detail at some of these later in the book.

And then there are the more secretive groups who hold private, invite-only meetings in exclusive locations around the world. They have names such as The Bilderburg Group (an annual meeting of high level people from the fields of energy, finance, government, intelligence, academia and the media), Skull & Bones (a secret society of elite seniors from Yale University), or the Committee of 300 (an organisation rumoured to include members from royal families, ex-heads of state and other wealthy and influential individuals).

A quick search on Google for any of these groups can quickly lead you down an endless rabbit warren of conjecture, mystery and paranoia.

Finally there are wealthy individuals who also have a big global influence through their network of connections and partnerships. Families like the Rockerfellers and Rothschilds have built deep generational wealth, which it is suggested has allowed them to keep a hand on the levers of control through the decades.

New wealth too can offer a seat at the mythical world elite table. Newly minted internet billionaires shape the lives we live – think of Jeff Bezos, and how Amazon has become a part of everyday life for millions of people. Mark Zuckerberg and Jack Dorsey, via Facebook and Twitter respectively, can shape our view of the world through the algorithms they build to feed us the content they think we want to see. They can also direct the current narrative by promoting some stories and censoring others. The suggestion is that we only see what they want us to see.

And let's not forget Bill Gates, philanthropic billionaire, who through The Bill and Melinda Gates Foundation, appears to be very enthusiastic about having us all immunised as soon as possible.

Are these the people who rule the world?

---

14 https://www.opec.org/opec_web/en/

15 https://www.weforum.org/

Do they have a cohesive plan for the future of mankind? Or are they simply bumbling along individually, like the rest of us, looking after their own affairs, hoping things will eventually turn out for the best?

What are your thoughts?

Do you think it's possible there is a secret cabal of global decision-makers who discuss and develop policies and plans behind closed doors that impact all of our lives in ways we can't quite see or understand?

It doesn't seem like a too farfetched conclusion to draw does it?

People with power and influence must certainly be interested in the future, and how as a global community we move forward. They must see the same global issues we all do, and feel a need to do something about it.

In reality, surely we all have a vested interest in how we face the future, how we use the finite resources available to us, and how we care for the world around us. After all, our children and grandchildren are the ones who will inherit the Earth we leave behind for them.

It makes sense that in today's modern, connected world, many of the problems we face need global solutions, and require action to be taken on a worldwide scale. These problems won't be fixed at government level of individual countries, as there can't really be a coordinated international solution without coordinated global leadership.

So let's go back to our childhood game of the imagination:

"If I ruled the world..."

What do you see as the biggest problems our world currently faces, aside from the obvious global pandemic, which we'll be coming to shortly, I promise?

- Climate change?
- Dwindling fossil fuel resources?
- Population growth?
- Poverty and hunger?
- Access to clean water and sanitation?
- Seemingly endless international war-mongering?
- Social and political division?
- The widening gap between rich and poor?
- Soaring rates of obesity and ill health?

This is by no means an exhaustive list of the issues we face together, all of which need resolving fairly soon, if we want our offspring to inherit a better world from us.

So it's probably safe to assume that these are the problems the global elites are working on – the same problems that would concern us if we held a similar position of power, wealth and influence.

> **NOTE:** I have used the term "global elite" here for the first time, for want of a better word, to mean anyone in a position of wealth and influence beyond a national level. Even this phrase can have an air of "conspiracy theory" about it, as if to even think of people making decisions with worldwide impact suggests you have joined the "flat-earthers" and "tin-foil hatters".
>
> As we'll discover throughout this journey of critical thought, it is becoming much easier to be so labelled when you start to question the overall narrative.

How would you, as ruler of the world, seek to address these problems? None of them have quick-fix easy answers, and all solutions will probably involve some sort of trade-off.

How would you address the problem of climate change? More renewable energy sources? Less carbon emissions? Nuclear power?

Do you see the continuous growth of the world population as a key issue? We're fast approaching 8 billion people. How do you control this unfettered growth without imposing draconian measures?

What about dwindling fossil fuels? Coal and oil have powered most of the world's development over the past couple of centuries. Can we continue to extract these resources from the ground to fuel endless expansion? Can new reserves be discovered and developed quickly enough to keep pace with a growing world population, all aspiring to "live the dream" of home and car ownership?

You can be pretty confident that these challenges, and solutions to them, occupy the thoughts of the global elite. It is almost certain that potential remedies for these issues are regularly discussed behind closed doors.

So let's get started on our journey of critical thinking by asking ourselves a few questions.

There aren't any right or wrong answers. The goal is simply to start the process of considering what we believe about how the world around us works. I certainly can't claim to know what the truth is. Possibly none of us ever will. But that doesn't mean we can ignore these matters, as we've already seen the dramatic impact the decisions made by others can have on our lives.

First of all, do you believe there is a group, or several groups, of companies, organisations and individuals at a level above national government, who make decisions that influence the future of the planet, and all of us who live on it?

If so, do you think these wealthy "global elites" have the best interests of the general global populace in mind when they consider their potential solutions?

Or perhaps you imagine that the ideas they come up with will be somewhat more self-serving?

The answer you come up with for this will colour most of what follows, and will have a significant impact on your view of how things are playing out, and what it all means.

Are you already convinced that our futures are being decided for us by people with very little concern for us "little people"?

Or maybe their intentions aren't bad, but the solutions they will be forced to implement will have dire consequences for us all?

Perhaps you're not so sure. It does all sound very conspiratorial, doesn't it?

There is nothing wrong at all with sitting on the fence, not sure of what is true and what isn't. In fact, as mentioned in Part 1, we'll be looking in more detail later in the book at the slippery nature of truth in today's media.

As I said in the introduction to this thought-provoking journey, I don't really know the answers to any of the questions this book raises. All we can do is consider the possibilities, weigh up the likelihood of something being true or not, and try to come to a considered opinion of how our world functions. Only then will we be able to make choices for ourselves, based on rational critical thinking, rather than taking the easy route of following the herd and doing exactly what we're told to do.

Maybe you think there couldn't possibly be a secretive cabal of global elites, working together to pull the strings of power from high above.

So if there is nobody at the top of the pyramid in control of things, who is steering the ship? Or are we just drifting towards disaster, without any guiding hand on the global tiller?

In that case we'll have to look to our individual governments for guidance in tough times. Let's take a look next at the politicians in whom we are forced to place our trust.

Our politicians

Why do people ever choose to become politicians? I couldn't ever imagine wanting such a role.

It seems that whatever choice you make, half the country will hate you for it, and you'll be harangued ceaselessly by the media. There is rarely a win-win solution for a political leader.

But there must be an appeal for many, as there is never a shortage of volunteers willing to step up and take on roles in government, or positions in the opposition parties.

I'm sure many idealistic bright youngsters hope they can make a big difference in the world, and see political office as a way to effect change for the better. But I also suspect there are many more who see politics as an easy option to cruise through their career, secure in a taxpayer funded position for life.

Perhaps one of the biggest draws is the lure of power – the power to make decisions that affect other people's lives. After all, that is a huge part of the political process... the endless tinkering with rules and regulations, taxes and tariffs.

A closer look at our political system, which we are endlessly told is a "democracy", reveals that in reality we have very little say over how our lives are run. We are offered a basic choice between two opposing parties, forced to choose between Option A or Option B at the ballot box. Of course there may be a third or fourth political party, but the majority of "democracies" boil down to a 2-horse race.

The spectacle of election offers us the illusion of choice, but the representatives of each party seem to spend more time trying to drag their opponents through the dirt than they do trying to consider which policies might be best for the constituents they are supposed to represent.

Ultimately it seems to matter little who gets voted in. Things remain much the same under the new party, a few minor changes of policy make little real difference, and we all go about our daily lives once more, just trying to get by as best we can.

This theatre of democratic free choice is easily called into question when in many cases the party that ends up in power does so by gaining less than half the votes cast.

So again, let's just take a moment to ask a few questions, and consider our opinions as we try to make sense in a world that seems to be unravelling around us.

QUESTION: What is your opinion of the politicians who run your country?

Here are a few possible answers.

- They're great! They have things under control, and we can all sleep peacefully at night, safe in the knowledge that they are hard at work building a better future for us.
- Generally they're doing the best job they can, and have our best interests at heart.
- They're probably mostly harmless, well-meaning managers of the day-to-day running of the country.
- They're incompetent idiots who couldn't organise the proverbial piss-up in a brewery.
- They are malignant overlords, using their positions of power to further their own interests, and we're just pawns in their bigger game.

Obviously your answer is going to be very personal, based on the country you live in, the people currently in power and your own personal political leanings.

QUESTION: How has your government acted since the coronavirus crisis began?

Once again, your answer will depend on many factors, including of course your own thoughts on how the current crisis should have been handled from the beginning.

Have your political leaders made good decisions, been clear in their communication, and fair in distribution of timely assistance to those in need? Or have their policies been slow, muddled, inconclusive, and full of U-turns?

QUESTION: Do you trust what your politicians tell you?

Are they impartial and is their main concern the safety and wellbeing of their constituents - you? Is everything they ask you to do, or mandate you do through bringing in new laws, for your eventual benefit?

Or are they perhaps more beholden to the pullers of the purse-strings, the lobbyists and those with deep pockets who fund political campaigns?

The World Health Organization (WHO)

The international body tasked with dealing with healthcare matters on a worldwide basis, including handling potential pandemic outbreaks, is the World Health Organization.

To say that their messaging was mixed throughout the early stages of the pandemic would be a bit of an understatement. And they have certainly received a lot of criticism for their handling of the crisis.

On 14th January 2020 a now infamous tweet[16] from the WHO stated:

> Preliminary investigations conducted by the Chinese authorities have found no clear evidence of human-to-human transmission of the novel #coronavirus (2019-nCoV) identified in #Wuhan, #China.

On 23rd January the WHO emergency committee couldn't reach a consensus on whether to classify the viral spread as a "Public Health Emergency of International Concern" (PHEIC).

> With final authority resting with the DG (Director-General), Tedros decided to wait despite admitting that "this is an emergency in China." A week later, he declared a PHEIC. By that point, confirmed cases of COVID-19 had increased tenfold with 7,781 cases across 18 countries.

The WHO definition[17] of the term 'pandemic' is "the worldwide spread of a new disease." At the end of January the virus was already spreading in at least 18 countries. It wasn't until almost 6 weeks later, on 11th March, that the WHO declared the outbreak a pandemic. By that time the virus "had killed more than 4,000 people, and had infected 118,000 people across nearly every continent."[18]

The WHO Director-General, Dr. Tedros Adhanom Ghebreyesus, was the focus of much attention, and an article published on 27th February 2020 on the Council on Foreign Relations website[19] criticized his apparent pro-China bias:

---

[16] https://twitter.com/WHO/status/1217043229427761152?s=20

[17] https://www.who.int/csr/disease/swineflu/frequently_asked_questions/pandemic/en/

[18] https://www.theatlantic.com/politics/archive/2020/04/world-health-organization-blame-pandemic-coronavirus/609820/

[19] https://www.cfr.org/blog/who-and-china-dereliction-duty

> On January 28, Tedros met with Chinese President Xi Jinping in Beijing. Following the meeting, Tedros commended China for "setting a new standard for outbreak control" and praised the country's top leadership for its "openness to sharing information" with the WHO and other countries.
>
> Yet in Wuhan, the epicenter of the COVID-19 outbreak, Chinese officials were busy arresting and punishing citizens for "spreading rumors" about the disease, while online censors controlled the flow of information.
>
> Despite growing evidence of China's mishandling of the outbreak and rising domestic Chinese outrage over the government's censorship, Tedros remains unmoved.
>
> On February 20 at the Munich Security Conference, Tedros doubled down on his praise for China stating that "China has bought the world time."

In April 2020 President Trump called for the withholding of United States funding for the WHO, criticizing them for mishandling the situation, resulting, he suggested, in worse outcomes.

"The reality is that the WHO failed to adequately obtain and share information in a timely and transparent fashion," he stated.

He accused the WHO of parroting misinformation pushed by the Chinese government which down-played the seriousness of the outbreak in the early days in Wuhan. The WHO's deference to China, Trump claimed, allowed the virus to spread internationally, resulting in thousands of unnecessary deaths.

This article on yahoo.com offers a balanced discussion on whether Trump's criticism is justified, or whether he was using the WHO as a scapegoat for his own errors of judgement:
https://news.yahoo.com/trumps-who-attacks-fair-criticism-or-scapegoating-150610957.html

This article in The Atlantic, referenced earlier, also provides a good overview of the criticisms levelled at the WHO:
https://www.theatlantic.com/politics/archive/2020/04/world-health-organization-blame-pandemic-coronavirus/609820/

What are your thoughts?

How much trust can we place in an organisation that seems to court so much controversy? Whose interests are they serving? How much faith can we put in them as the organisation at the forefront of the push "to make sure COVID-19 vaccines can be safely delivered to all those who need them"?[20]

From the WHO COVID-19 vaccines page:
https://www.who.int/emergencies/diseases/novel-coronavirus-2019/covid-19-vaccines

> The world is in the midst of a COVID-19 pandemic. As WHO and partners work together on the response - tracking the pandemic, advising on critical interventions, distributing vital medical supplies to those in need - they are racing to develop and deploy safe and effective vaccines.

It is interesting to note that on this page of the WHO website, among all of the glowingly positive vaccine information, there is a section filled with links to articles dedicated to "combating misinformation", with titles such as:

- Let's flatten the infodemic curve
- Latest trusted updates on each COVID-19 vaccine in development
- Report misinformation about COVID-19
- Mythbusters
- Responsible media reporting on COVID-19 Vaccines

How do you feel the WHO has conducted itself from the beginning of the viral outbreak? Did they act quickly and decisively? How about their messaging... has it been clear, concise and effective?

How are they doing with on-going pandemic management?

Is their pro-vaccine messaging based on their belief that this is the only way out of the problem we currently face?

---

[20] https://www.who.int/emergencies/diseases/novel-coronavirus-2019/covid-19-vaccines

National health organisations

In the USA there is a veritable alphabet soup of government bodies involved with health, medicine and food.

Here is the basic structure of the Department of Health and Human Services (HHS)[21], a cabinet-level department which includes the following agencies:

1) Centers for Disease Control and Prevention (CDC)
    a) National Institute for Occupational Safety and Health (NIOSH)
    b) Coordinating Center for Infectious Diseases (CCID)
        i) National Center for Preparedness, Detection, and Control of Infectious Diseases (NCPDCID)
            (1) Division of Healthcare Quality Promotion (DHQP)
    c) Healthcare Infection Control Practices Advisory Committee (HICPAC)
2) Centers for Medicare and Medicaid Services (CMS)
3) National Institutes of Health (NIH)
    a) The National Institute of Allergy and Infectious Diseases (NIAID)
    b) National Library of Medicine (NLM)
4) Food and Drug Administration (FDA)
5) Health Resources and Services Administration (HRSA)
6) Agency for Healthcare Research and Quality (AHRQ)

Several of these agencies appear regularly in news and discussions about the pandemic. CDC, FDA, NIH and NIAID are probably acronyms you're much more familiar with at the start of 2021 than you were a year ago.

In the UK, news reports generally refer to Public Health England (PHE). From the UK Government website[22], "What Public Health England does: We exist to protect and improve the nation's health and wellbeing, and reduce health inequalities. PHE is an executive agency, sponsored by the Department of Health and Social Care."

"What the Department of Health and Social Care does: We support ministers in leading the nation's health and social care to help people live

---

[21] https://apic.org/Resource_/TinyMceFileManager/Advocacy-PDFs/outline_of_govt_health_agencies.pdf

[22] https://www.gov.uk/government/organisations/public-health-england

more independent, healthier lives for longer. DHSC is a ministerial department, supported by 29 agencies and public bodies."[23]

There is an equally bewildering array of government agencies and think tanks with catchy acronyms and slightly vague descriptions of their responsibilities. Here are a couple of regularly featured favourites on the UK national news:

> NERVTAG (The New and Emerging Respiratory Virus Threats Advisory Group)[24]
>
> SAGE (Scientific Advisory Group for Emergencies)[25]

How do you feel your government agencies are doing? Is your hard-earned tax dollar or tax pound being well spent?

---

[23] https://www.gov.uk/government/organisations/department-of-health-and-social-care

[24] https://www.gov.uk/government/groups/new-and-emerging-respiratory-virus-threats-advisory-group

[25] https://www.gov.uk/government/organisations/scientific-advisory-group-for-emergencies

The media

The way we consume "news" in the 21st Century is very different to how we received information on current events before the internet was a part of our everyday lives.

TV News used to be on a couple of times each evening. In the UK, on the trusted BBC, there was a 6 o'clock program, another at 9pm, and if you stayed up long enough, a late night summary of events. The other main sources of information were either the daily newspaper, which was already out of date by a day when you bought it, or the radio.

Today there is a huge range of 24-hour-a-day TV news sources, available on demand from around the world, with up-to-the-minute reports of events from all continents. This is supplemented by an endless range of online services too, which provide instant access to almost real-time coverage of unfolding issues.

Competition is fierce for "eyeballs" on the screen, and so the line between news and entertainment can become blurred. With so many hours of airtime to fill, and content to provide, much of the "news" is geared to not only impartial information, but to opinion, debate, and infotainment. Also worth mentioning are the numerous paid-for and sponsored posts you'll find interspersed with your daily "factual" news articles.

But despite this huge range of services, the number of people who control the flow of information is surprisingly small. In the USA there are 6 major corporations, often referred to as "The Big 6", who collectively control almost all U.S. media. These companies are Time Warner, Walt Disney, Viacom, Rupert Murdoch's News Corp, CBS Corporation and GE.

According to one of the fascinating graphics on this page, "In 1983 90% of America's news media was owned by 50 different companies. In 2011, the same 90% was owned by just these 6 companies."
https://gizmodo.com/fascinating-graphic-shows-who-owns-all-the-major-brands-1599537576

The fact that our news is fed to us from the same limited sources is clearly evidenced in video montages from different news stations across the country, when presenters talk about the same subject, using exactly the same words.

Simply search YouTube for the term "Newscasters agree" and you'll find plenty of examples. Many of these montages seem fairly harmless, covering "local news issues" such as the Easter Bunny, or online shopping sales.

But things take on a bit more of a sinister feel when the messaging is clearly designed to sway public opinion, as in this disturbing and dystopian montage:
https://www.youtube.com/watch?v=_fHfgU8oMSo

Social media

It is beyond doubt that social media has its darker side, and is a cause for concern for many reasons. It is suggested that rather than making us happier, seeing the edited and air-brushed highlights of the lives of our friends online makes us feel that our lives are lessened by comparison.

Social media platforms also seem to support the bitter resentful side that hides inside many people, and so-called "trolls" can be found anywhere there is an opportunity to have an opinion.

The divisive nature of social media is highlighted and explained in a very enlightening Netflix documentary called "The Social Dilemma".[26]

The business model most social platforms embrace is to give people a free forum for communication and entertainment. The companies make their income by selling advertising space to businesses who want to be seen by the millions, or billions of users. Therefore, the main aim of social networks is to keep people engaged with their screen as long as possible, to show them as many adverts as possible.

To do this the platforms build algorithms – automated computer software – designed to watch your every move online, then figure out exactly what interests you, aiming to feed you more of the content you like, with the ultimate goal of keeping your attention. The outcome of this is that you receive a very personalised feed.

If, for example, you show a great interest in UFOs, with a slant towards believing they exist, your feed will become more populated with people and information supporting your belief. If on the other hand you show great scepticism about UFOs, you'll have a very different online experience.

It is easy to see how this can result in wide divides of opinion. When this example is applied to political leanings, or any other divisive topic, such as the UK's recent Brexit debacle, you don't need to look much further to understand how our society has become so divided and intolerant.

What are your feelings about social media? Are you a regular user? Do you consider it to be a reliable source of information on current affairs? Do you feel that the articles you see in your feed offer a balanced and impartial view of the world?

No judgement is intended here, this is just an exercise in being more conscious about the sources we use to gather information, upon which we base our opinions. Ultimately it is these opinions which help us make the decisions which shape our future.

---

[26] https://www.imdb.com/title/tt11464826/

Big Pharma

Can Big Pharma be trusted?

We'll look in much more detail at the pharmaceutical industry in the next section. But for now, just remember that these are the very companies that we're going to be trusting if we decide to roll up our sleeves to receive one of the new vaccines.

Is our health their number one priority?

Here are just a few articles, and a few quotes, produced by a quick search for the term "can big pharma be trusted":

From Aljazeera[27]:

ARTICLE: Big Pharma is not willing to help us defeat COVID-19

> There have already been attempts to design a system which can help the world provide coronavirus medicines which would be available to all on a fair basis. Costa Rica proposed allowing countries and researchers to share their technologies, collaborate on research and produce patent-free medicines back in the spring.
>
> Despite gaining broad support from around the world, Big Pharma howled in protest. Pfizer called it "nonsense". British companies working on coronavirus treatments, AstraZeneca and GlaxoSmithKlein, refused to participate, backed by the British government which tried to water down the proposals. When asked whether he would attend the launch of the Costa Rican scheme, the director of a prominent Big Pharma lobbying group, said he was 'too busy'.

It is interesting to note that this article was published on 18th October 2020, before either Pfizer or AstraZenica, both mentioned in the article, announced their new vaccine trial successes.

Law firm Beasley Allen came out close to the top of the search results list, with a December 2019 feature[28]:

---

[27] https://www.aljazeera.com/opinions/2020/10/18/big-pharma-is-not-going-to-help-the-world-defeat-covid-19/

[28] https://www.beasleyallen.com/news/leading-medical-journal-says-big-pharma-cannot-be-trusted/

ARTICLE: Leading medical journal says Big Pharma cannot be trusted

The lead paragraph reads:

> In a scathing editorial published this month, leading medical journal BMJ went toe-to-toe with Big Pharma, arguing that industry-sponsored clinical trials for major drugs and medical devices are "causing harm" to consumers, because they are more likely to find favorable results. Instead, the journal opined, governments should fund independent trials for a more unbiased and trustworthy result.

On the same first page of search results The Sydney Morning Herald features a story[29] about the same BMJ article:

ARTICLE: 'Cannot be trusted ... causing harm': Top medical journal takes on big pharma

> The BMJ says doctors are being unduly influenced by industry-sponsored education events and industry-funded trials for major drugs.
>
> Those trials cannot be trusted, the journal's editor and a team of global healthcare leaders write in a scathing editorial published on Wednesday.
>
> The "endemic financial entanglement with industry is distorting the production and use of healthcare evidence, causing harm to individuals and waste for health systems", they write.

Unfortunately neither the Beasley Allen article nor SMH article has a link to the original BMJ article they quote. A quick search on the BMJ site for the direct quote in the SMH article soon turns up the BMJ original here:
https://www.bmj.com/content/367/bmj.l6576

Finally, here's an article from Harvard University's Center For Ethics[30], which although aiming its criticism more at the FDA (U.S. Food and Drug Administration), it reflects on the products sold by the big pharma companies.

---

[29] https://www.smh.com.au/national/cannot-be-trusted-causing-harm-top-medical-journal-takes-on-big-pharma-20191203-p53ggj.html

[30] https://ethics.harvard.edu/blog/risky-drugs-why-fda-cannot-be-trusted

ARTICLE: Risky Drugs: Why The FDA Cannot Be Trusted

> The bar for 'safe' is equally low, and over the past 30 years, approved drugs have caused an epidemic of harmful side effects, even when properly prescribed. Every week, about 53,000 excess hospitalizations and about 2400 excess deaths occur in the United States among people taking properly prescribed drugs to be healthier. One in every five drugs approved ends up causing serious harm...

Just go back and read that quote from the Harvard Uni article again.

"Every week ... about 2400 excess deaths occur ... among people taking properly prescribed drugs" made by the same companies who are now trying to convince us their hastily produced vaccines, currently administered in the USA under Emergency Use Authorization only (more on this later), are desirable, safe and effective.

What are your thoughts on the priorities of Big Pharma companies?

Our medical professionals

It has been widely reported that doctors and hospitals in the States have been financially incentivised to categorise people as COVID patients.

Categorising a patient as a COVID-19 case attracts a payment to the hospital from the U.S. government of USD $13,000. If the patient ends up on a ventilator the sum paid is three times as much, at $39,000.

FactCheck.org gives further details on how this information emerged, and the response to it[31]:

ARTICLE: Hospital Payments and the COVID-19 Death Count

> The initial comment [about hospitals deliberately miscoding patients] was made by Minnesota State Sen. Scott Jensen, a family physician, who spoke with Fox News host Laura Ingraham on April 8 about the idea that the number of COVID-19 deaths may be inflated. Jensen was responding to National Institute of Allergy and Infectious Diseases Director Anthony Fauci, who — while answering a reporter's question about that theory — said "you will always have conspiracy theories when you have very challenging public health crises. They are nothing but distractions."
>
> Jensen, April 8: "I would remind him [Fauci] that anytime health care intersects with dollars it gets awkward. Right now Medicare has determined that if you have a COVID-19 admission to the hospital, you'll get paid $13,000. If that COVID-19 patient goes on a ventilator, you get $39,000, three times as much. Nobody can tell me after 35 years in the world of medicine that sometimes those kinds of things impact on what we do.
>
> In an interview with FactCheck.org, however, Jensen said he did not think that hospitals were intentionally misclassifying cases for financial reasons.
>
> But that's how his comments have been widely interpreted and paraded on social media. One YouTube video with Jensen's interview, viewed 42,000 times, was titled "US: Hospitals Get Paid More to List Patients as COVID-19"

The video to which FactCheck refers should be available at this link: https://www.youtube.com/watch?v=DsLsHqoz5eU

---

31 https://www.factcheck.org/2020/04/hospital-payments-and-the-covid-19-death-count/

Unfortunately, the YouTube censors have been at work, and all that can be seen there now is a black-screen "Video unavailable" notice.

This may be the interview video the article intended to link to, still available elsewhere on YouTube at time of going to print. It makes interesting viewing:
https://www.youtube.com/watch?v=_qWmiWf81zI

Our peers

It seems that our world has become more divided and fractious than ever over the past few years. American politics divides the nation into two bitterly opposed camps of ardent supporters of their own side.

Trump's surprise election win in 2016 gave the USA one of their most controversial presidents ever. The 2020 election is widely considered to be one of the most divisive and bitter political contests in recent history.

The Brexit vote in 2016, when a British referendum called on the populace to decide on whether the UK should leave the European Union, caused many bitter rivalries between old friends, and often within families. Passions ran high on both sides of the debate.

The whole messy debacle continued for a further 4 years as bungling politicians failed to reach any agreement time and time again, frittering away millions of pounds of taxpayer money in the process.

Social media continues to offer a voice for the trolls who seem to want to rant and rave about anything and everything.

Black Lives Matter, sexual identity, #MeToo, cancel culture, Antifa, Yellow Jackets, the Twitter Mob, and political correctness have filled our collective conscience.

This background of widely divided opinion, and lack of tolerance for others who hold a different viewpoint, coupled with the pressure-cooker of stress created by fears of a virus, lockdowns and uncertainty about our financial future, all put extra strain upon our personal relationships.

Any discussion of the pandemic, masks, lockdowns, government response, medical options and vaccines can quickly escalate into strong disagreement, or worse.

It seems that our current dilemma is just as divisive as all that has gone before over the past few years. If you express your discomfort at the idea of taking a vaccine which has been pushed through in record time, it is quite possible you will be branded as selfishly endangering the lives of others.

On the other hand if you decide the vaccine is in your best interest, and you're willing to accept the trade-off of haste vs. getting back to a more normal life, you can quickly find yourself ridiculed as a sheep, following along without questioning or thinking.

One would think there was some reasonable middle ground for those of us who wish to invest some time in researching, thinking about and questioning what is going on before we jump to a hasty decision with little or no consideration.

Unfortunately, it seems that just questioning the narrative in any way can get you labelled as a "conspiracy theorist" by those on one side of the fence, who believe your reluctance to be vaccinated endangers other people's lives. Those who firmly believe beyond a shadow of a doubt that there are evil goings-on in the shadows will mock your wavering uncertainty, branding you as "naive" for not embracing the darkest of possibilities.

In today's deeply divided world even the Goldilocks sweet-spot in the middle, halfway between unquestioning complacency and deep paranoia, can sometimes draw its own degree of criticism from our peers.

PART 3:
THE ASSUMPTIONS WE MAKE

"Never ASSUME, because when you ASSUME, you make an ASS of U and ME."

Anonymous

Making an ass out of u and me

In order to reach a decision point on taking, or not taking, a vaccine, we need to consider the assumptions we may, or may not, be making, consciously or sub-consciously, as we consider our questions, opinions and conclusions.

We'll look at these assumptions by grouping them in four broad categories:

1. People, businesses and organisations
2. The virus, testing and numbers
3. Lockdowns and the economy
4. Vaccines and outcomes

People / Businesses / Organisations

We'll begin by taking a look at some of the assumptions we might (or might not) be making about the people, businesses and organisations involved in the current crisis, and particularly in the roll-out of the vaccines which are deemed necessary to get us out of this situation.

People in general are good

Most people are pretty decent. Most of us just want to get on with building the best life we can for ourselves and our families. We're prepared to help and support others to the best of our ability when we can.

The world is a competitive place, and as such we do have to compete with others, for example, to win the partner we desire, for the job we want, the house we plan to buy, or any other limited resources we wish to acquire. But generally we manage to do all of this by imposing minimal harm on others.

Most of us (hopefully) wouldn't entertain the idea of doing deliberate harm to others to get ahead.

This is why it is so hard for most people to accept that there are others in our society who are different. There are those who have less of a conscience, and are willing to deceive, steal, and even kill to get what they want.

For most of us the only time we cross paths with this kind of mindset is in the movies, or perhaps when we become the unfortunate victim of such a person.

Our "decency bias" means that it is almost impossible for us to imagine what goes on in the mind of a serial killer, or a murderous despot. We can't really comprehend how people like Hitler, Stalin, Pinochet or Ceausescu[32] think, and how they can be responsible for millions of deaths, but appear to show little remorse.

We're shocked when we hear about how the tobacco industry continued to fight their corner for decades when it became obvious their product was responsible for thousands of deaths. Their obvious motive was to keep the huge profits rolling in.

We're disgusted when a company pollutes a water source with toxic runoff, simply because it is cheaper and easier than to deal with their waste products in a responsible manner. It can take years to uncover such

---

[32] https://historycollection.com/10-cruel-despotic-leaders-20th-century/

transgressions, and in the meantime thousands who use that water source develop cancer and die.

Perhaps it is easier for the executives in these positions to act in this way because they are one step removed from the death and misery they inflict on others in the name of corporate profit. They don't have to look their victim in the eye as they pull a trigger. I wonder how they sleep at night? It is hard for a decent person to imagine that there are people who behave in this way, and sleep soundly, untroubled by their conscience.

Our politicians are often forced to make life-and-death decisions. Does the killing of a wanted terrorist warrant a drone strike at a wedding gathering? Again, it is hard for us to imagine a leader taking a decision like this without having a sleepless night afterwards.

There is also a mountain of evidence that others less malevolent are still willing to commit atrocities when under the influence or power of a less principled leader. "I was just following orders" is a commonly heard defence for many unspeakable acts.

This decency bias that most of us have makes it so easy to denounce the more nightmarish scenarios suggested for what may be happening around us as "conspiracy theories".

It is too much for us to believe, for example, that a worldwide vaccination program could actually be a mass-sterilization program designed to halt the rampant, unsustainable population growth that is overwhelming our planet's natural systems.

Ridiculous. Nobody could possibly be that evil. That's just conspiracy theory nonsense!

> **NOTE:** I'm not suggesting this is actually the case for our current crisis. I merely use this as an example to illustrate how easy it is to discount such theories, as they are so far beyond our ability to conceive as possible. However, it is exactly this inability to believe such suggestions that allowed leaders like Hitler, Stalin, Pinochet or Ceausescu to gain power and inflict their atrocities.

Our leaders are selfless

In an earlier chapter we looked at the people we trust, and wondered about the reasons a person might seek out a position in political office.

We would all hope that the people we elect to make decisions on our behalf are there because they really do have the interests of the nation at heart. They aspire to these positions because they "want to serve".

Indeed, we refer to people who hold government positions either by election or appointment as "public servants". This loaded term[33] suggests that our government is there to serve the public.

However, we're all motivated by self-interest to a significant degree, and to think otherwise about those who aspire to positions of power would be naive, to say the least.

Whose interests do most politicians really serve?

Maybe the answer lies in the never ending news stories of political scandal, back-stabbing, lies and deceit, mis-appropriation of funds, acceptance of bribes, and general political grift.

The media is honest and impartial

I'm not quite sure where to begin with this section. If I need to convince you that most of the mainstream media sources who feed us our worldview are influenced, biased, deceitful and corrupt, than I'm amazed you've made it this far into the book without throwing it aside.

Controlling influence over TV, newspapers, magazines and online news sources has been concentrated over the past decades into fewer and fewer hands.

As we saw in the previous chapter, 90% of U.S. media sources in 1983 were owned by 50 different companies. By 2011 90% of media was owned and run by just 6.

If you didn't watch the video linked from the earlier section about the media I encourage you to do so now:
https://www.youtube.com/watch?v=_fHfgU8oMSo

It is amazing to see more than 30 different news anchors at Sinclair-owned local news stations parroting an identical script which apparently warns us, without a hint of irony, that there is a "troubling trend of irresponsible, one-sided news stories plaguing our country."

Apparently, "this is extremely dangerous to our democracy".

Honest and impartial? You decide.

Social media is unbiased and uncensored

In the previous section we looked at how AI (Artificial Intelligence) algorithms used by social media companies skew what you see in your

---

33 https://www.thefreedictionary.com/public+servant

personal feed, providing you with a very personalized and unique view of the world. As the documentary The Social Dilemma suggested, this isn't necessarily malignant in design, but is merely aimed at keeping your eyeballs on the screen for longer.

But is there a more conscious manipulation of what we see via our social media platforms?

There have certainly been many, many acts of censorship, as articles, comments and videos questioning the main narrative, or offering alternative theories for what is happening around us, have been deleted.

Facebook and Twitter have both been active in deleting content that they label as dangerous misinformation, or that "violates company policies". The 2020 election caused much discussion of the reach and influence social media platforms have in deciding what people see.[34] It isn't too hard to imagine that there may be a hidden, or not so hidden, agenda supported by social media platforms, as promoted by the interviewee in this article.[35]

ARTICLE: Post-2020 election, Covid vaccine is biggest disinformation threat on the internet: Former Facebook security chief

> "When you talk about vaccines ... there will be very complicated, conflicting information and we need information centers equivalent to what we had running for the election," Stamos said. "Facebook should set the goal of four million people getting vaccinated that wouldn't otherwise, just like they registered four million," he said.

YouTube, owned by Google, have also been hard at work silencing voices who speak out against the common narrative. In order for videos to avoid being banned, or de-monetized[36], video creators have had to avoid even mentioning the word "coronavirus", using euphemistic terminology such as "WuFlu" or "cerveza sickness".

---

[34] https://www1.cbn.com/cbnnews/us/2020/june/facebook-announces-new-censorship-plan-as-employees-reveal-their-anti-conservative-anti-trump-agenda

[35] https://www.cnbc.com/2020/10/31/2020-election-coronavirus-vaccine-disinformation-will-continue.html

[36] https://www.theverge.com/2020/3/4/21164553/youtube-coronavirus-demonetization-sensitive-subjects-advertising-guidelines-revenue

YouTube's "COVID-19 Medical Misinformation Policy"[37] states:

> YouTube doesn't allow content that spreads medical misinformation that contradicts local health authorities' or the World Health Organization's (WHO) medical information about COVID-19. This is limited to content that contradicts WHO or local health authorities' guidance on:
>
> - Treatment
> - Prevention
> - Diagnostic
> - Transmission

Well thank you YouTube for keeping us safe from any opinion that contradicts WHO.

Google, YouTube's parent company, has hardly been impartial in how it presents information to us.

I have to give full credit here to John Iovine, author of the book Scamdemic[38], for his eye-opening information on how Google manipulates and skews the search predictions we see when typing our queries into the Google search bar.

In Google's own words, the goal of the auto-complete function of their search bar is to predict what you are about to type, in order to get you to the results of your search as quickly as possible. They are keen to point out that they are not offering suggestions, merely basing their prediction of where you're heading, based on search term popularity and current trending searches.

Therefore we can assume from their statement that they want us to believe they are not trying to influence or misdirect us in any way. They want us to find exactly what we are looking for as quickly as possible. Here's their explanation[39] of this function:

> When you start a search on Google, you can quickly find info with search predictions. Search predictions are possible search terms related to what you're looking for **and what other people have already searched for**.

---

[37] https://support.google.com/youtube/answer/9891785?hl=en

[38] https://www.amazon.com/Scamdemic-COVID-19-Agenda-Liberals-White-ebook/dp/B08DHMYQNK

[39] https://support.google.com/websearch/answer/106230

> Google makes search predictions based on factors, like **popularity or similarity**. When you choose a prediction, you do a search using the term you selected.
>
> Important: You can't turn off search predictions. Search predictions are built into Google Search to help you find information faster and easier. You can always choose not to click on a suggestion from search predictions. [emphasis added]

John then runs through an example of how this function shows obvious bias in what it offers you as "popular or similar".

His example is a search for the term "do vaccines cause autism".

Try it now on google.com. Put in a search for "do vaccines c" and see what you are offered. On my screen the list of options include "do vaccines contain" with several further choices, "do vaccines create" and "do vaccines cause".

If we continue, and type our phrase as far as "do vaccines cause", I only see two predictions: "do vaccines cause herd immunity" and "do vaccines cause genetic mutations".

Adding "aut" to our search produces a top prediction of "do vaccines cause autoimmune flares".

Seriously? Is that searched for more times than "do vaccines cause autism"? Let's have a look.

From Google Trends[40] it would appear that our original search term has a weekly volume (USA) of anywhere between 0 and 100 searches. I'd guess the average to be around 40 per week. Seems low, but OK, let's go with that...

Apparently the term "do vaccines cause autoimmune flares" has no search data at all.
https://trends.google.com/trends/explore?geo=US&q=do%20vaccines%20cause%20autoimmune%20flares

> Hmm, your search doesn't have enough data to show here. Please make sure everything is spelled correctly, or try a more general term.

And yet Google "predicts" this is the term I am typing. If I continue to type, and add the letter "i", so that I now have the search "do vaccines

[40] https://trends.google.com/trends/explore?geo=US&q=do%20vaccines%20cause%20autism

cause auti", Google has nothing. No idea. Not a clue what I might be about to finish typing.

Once I complete the term and hit the search button I am notified by Google that there are over 5 million results for the search term. Top of the list is an article named "Do vaccines cause autism?" on the HistoryOfVaccines.org website. The page link also uses the same term in the URL:
https://www.historyofvaccines.org/index.php/content/articles/do-vaccines-cause-autism

The History Of Vaccines website is "an educational resource by The College of Physicians of Philadelphia". The article itself offers a balanced discussion of the topic, and cites 30 references after their conclusion that there is no conclusive evidence to link autism to vaccinations. Hardly the stuff of "tin foil hat" conspiracy theories, is it?

The HistoryOfVaccines page was last updated on 25th January 2018, so it has been online and unchanged for at least 3 years.

Strange, isn't it, that this page has a title that exactly matches the term I'm searching for, has the term built into the URL, has been online for over 3 years, and is the top result from over 5 million results Google could find for that term, and yet Google thinks a search term with no search volume data at all is a better prediction for what I was typing?

You'd almost think they wanted to divert me away from the search I was planning to make, wouldn't you?

Do you really think social media is unbiased and uncensored?

The pharma companies are concerned about our health

I don't think I am going to have to do too much digging to convince you that pharma companies tend to put their financial interests above those of the people they are meant to be treating and curing. If my digging doesn't convince you, at least I should be able to sew a few seeds of doubt.

In the articles below, look particularly for the companies currently involved in creating and distributing coronavirus vaccines. Past history is usually a good indicator of motivations for current actions.

From USA Today[41]:

[41] https://usatoday.com/story/news/investigations/2019/08/07/biologic-drug-makers-pay-doctors-prescriptions/1943331001/

ARTICLE: A surge in risky, expensive drug prescriptions: What's behind it? Millions from drugmakers.

> In 2011, a group of influential dermatologists – most with financial ties to drug companies – put out national guidelines for treating psoriasis.
>
> They said immune-suppressing drugs of a certain class could clear up mild skin issues before weddings and other special events.
>
> The problem: The recommendation went against approved uses for such drugs, which carry strict safety warnings from the U.S. Food and Drug Administration.

Here's a second example from the same article:

> In 2012, the drugmaker AbbVie created a "Nurse Ambassador" program that paid nurses around the country to visit patients with prescriptions for Humira, its rheumatoid arthritis and psoriasis drug.
>
> The wrinkle: Nurses were told not to mention the drug's risks, including potentially deadly infections, according to a lawsuit filed by California regulators.

Again, from the same article, **here's Pfizer**, one of the big names in the current vaccine roll-out:

> In 2014, **Pfizer** paid for a study of its rheumatoid arthritis drug Xeljanz – one authored by **12 experts, all with financial ties to the company**. Xeljanz came out on top.
>
> The twist: They didn't compare Xeljanz to the treatment considered most effective by experts.

The conclusion:

> All three efforts were part of **a massive drug company push to boost sales of expensive drugs** to treat autoimmune conditions such as psoriasis and rheumatoid arthritis.
>
> The drugs were introduced two decades ago and have hit **$45 billion in sales, despite escalating prices and mounting reports of serious side effects**...
>
> "There are a lot of different playbooks on drugs," said Diana Zuckerman, president of the Washington, D.C.-based National Center for Health Research, a patient advocacy group. **"The industry knows how to sell a product."** [emphasis added]

From a 2015 article on BusinessInsider.com[42]:

ARTICLE: These Are The Drugs Doctors Get Paid The Most To Promote

> Companies pay doctors millions of dollars to promote not their most innovative or effective drugs, but some of their most unremarkable.
>
> In the last five months of 2013, drug makers spent almost $20 million trying to convince physicians and teaching hospitals to give their freshly-patented drugs to patients, but many of them are near-copies of existing drugs that treat the same conditions.
>
> A hefty portion are also available as generics, chemically identical copies that work just as well at a fraction of the price. And still others have serious side effects that only became apparent after they were approved by the FDA.

Oh dear! From the same article, here's COVID vaccine manufacturer **AstraZenica**:

> Take multinational pharmaceutical company AstraZeneca's blood-thinning drug Brilinta, for example, ranked third in ProPublica's list[43] of the highest payments to doctors. One of Brilinta's biggest competitors, Plavix, has been available generically since 2012 at a fraction of the price.
>
> In order to make a profit in such a crowded market, producers of new drugs — who have often spent a fortune on research and development — must make them appealing to the doctors who prescribe them. A study published by Ornstein and Jones in March found that doctors often accept thousands of dollars in speaking and consulting payments from drug companies that also sponsor their research.
>
> During the last five months of 2013 (the period that Ornstein and Jones looked at for their most recent report), **Brilinta's manufacturers [AstraZenica] made 63 payments to doctors, totalling $282,000 in consulting fees**. [emphasis added]

---

[42] https://www.businessinsider.com/what-drugs-are-doctors-paid-the-most-to-promote-2015-1

[43] https://projects.propublica.org/docdollars/

I could go on, and on, and on... the two articles quoted above are picked from the first page of results for a search for the term "doctors paid to prescribe certain drugs", and already we've got damning evidence against two of the major manufacturers of the first batch of vaccines off the production line.

Not very encouraging, is it?

The Business Insider article above links a page titled "Dollars For Docs" on the website ProPublica.com, which has some fascinating info on drug company payments. They say, "Pharmaceutical and medical device companies are required by law to release details of their payments to a variety of doctors and U.S. teaching hospitals for promotional talks, research and consulting, among other categories."

The latest information on this page[44] details payments made in 2018. Pfizer Inc and AstraZenica Pharmaceuticals LP put in strong performances, in 9th and 10th position on the list, with payouts for the year of USD $48.9million and USD $45million respectively.

I imagine that kind of budget buys some serious influence.

Digging into the details shows that in 2018 **Pfizer made payments to 113,240 different doctors**. The top two doctors on this long list received payments totalling over $1.5million. They both work at the same place in Boston, Massachusetts. They are named on the website.[45]

AstraZenica were similarly magnanimous in 2018, handing out payments to over 84,000 different doctors. The top recipient alone received a whopping $1.47million that year.[46]

I wonder if these two companies are using any of the millions of dollars they have available in their annual budgets to buy influence in order to promote their latest new products to our care-givers?

Where do you think their 2020 and 2021 promotional budgets will be directed?

---

44 https://projects.propublica.org/docdollars/

45 https://projects.propublica.org/docdollars/company/100000000286

46 https://projects.propublica.org/docdollars/company/100000000146

Our health care systems look after us

We refer to "health care systems" when we think about the network of institutions we turn to when we are ill. A more accurate term might be "sick care systems".

In reality these institutions don't interest themselves as much in keeping us healthy, as they do in treating us when we are ill. There is no profit to be extracted from the wallets of those who stay healthy through a common sense approach to life combining good diet and plenty of exercise.

As Dr. Vernon Coleman, in his book "Vaccines Are Dangerous – And Don't Work[47]", says:

> Proper preventive medicine (persuading people to avoid really bad habits and to live a healthy lifestyle) is always difficult to sell to politicians, doctors and journalists because you cannot see the people who have been saved.
>
> Where is the evidence that something has been done?
>
> And more important where is the profit?

Our doctors give us the best advice they can

You're probably a little sceptical about our doctors already, if you read the "pharma" section above. You are probably right to be a little concerned. I'll refer you once more to the ProPublica website[48], which reveals the top pharma-paid doctor raked in $29million in 2018, 87 payments from 6 different pharma companies.[49]

You can look up any U.S. doctor on the website and see how he fares on this alarming league table of big pharma incentivisation.

As we discussed in the "people we trust" section, most doctors probably begin their journey into the medical profession with the best intentions. But along the way it is quite possible that financial incentives cause a lowering of moral values. Here are a few more quotes from articles produced by the same search term used in the "pharma companies" section above... "doctors paid to prescribe certain drugs":

---

47 https://www.amazon.com/Vaccines-Are-Dangerous-Dont-Work-ebook/dp/B00HSSRK1E/

48 https://projects.propublica.org/docdollars/

49 https://projects.propublica.org/docdollars/doctors/pid/311622

From the health section of USnews.com[50]

ARTICLE: Do Drug Company Payments to Doctors Influence Which Drugs They Prescribe?

> Although most doctors are incredibly honest, ethical people who only want to help patients, physicians are human and potentially vulnerable to influence from outside. Money is a prime suspect for undue influence, and it's probably no surprise that pharmaceutical companies spend billions annually to influence physicians and other drug prescribers to write more prescriptions for their particular products.
>
> Pharmaceutical marketing goes well beyond the half dozen commercials you might see during the nightly news. Ian Larkin, associate professor at the UCLA Anderson School of Management, has researched how pharmaceutical companies influence doctors' prescribing habits, and says that much of the marketing budget for many of these companies is directed towards direct contact with doctors. "Pharmaceutical companies are spending something like double the amount that they spend on research and development [of new drugs] on marketing to doctors." He says this is completely separate from the advertisements that we see on TV. That kind of marketing to consumers accounts for "only about 20 percent" of how much these companies spend on marketing their drugs, he says.

From healthline.com[51]:

ARTICLE: Is Your Doctor Getting Paid to Prescribe You Pain Relievers?

> In May [2019], a federal jury found top executives of the opioid manufacturer Insys Therapeutics guilty of racketeering charges related to the opioid epidemic.
>
> The criminal charges and guilty verdicts were a rarity, as it held high-ranking corporate officials responsible for bribing doctors to prescribe their fentanyl-based Subsys and intentionally misleading

---

[50] https://health.usnews.com/health-care/patient-advice/articles/2018-08-31/do-drug-company-payments-to-doctors-influence-which-drugs-they-prescribe

[51] https://www.healthline.com/health-news/is-your-doctor-getting-paid-to-prescribe-painkillers-for-you

> insurers of patients' needs for the potent and addictive pain reliever, as reported by The New York Times.
>
> Subsys was approved for use in cancer patients, but was soon prescribed for people with other problems like back pain, opening them up to potentially life-altering or life-ending opioid addictions. Medical experts, as well as federal authorities, say top-down pressure from executives at opioid-making drug companies helped fuel the opioid epidemic.
>
> According to the U.S. Centers for Disease Control and Prevention (CDC), the first wave of the opioid crisis — which kills an average of 130 people daily in the United States — first started in the 1990s when doctors began prescribing more opioids.

Government bureaucracy

Another factor to consider when looking at the advice our doctors give is the layers of government bureaucracy under which they must labour.

Here's Dr. Simone Gold from her book "I Do Not Consent"[52]:

> The real problem is the gradual intrusion of big government into the doctor-patient relationship, adding impossible and conflicting paperwork, red tape, and insoluble obstructions without improving the quality of care for the people I meet in hospital emergency rooms.

Do we always get the best advice possible from our doctors?

What are your thoughts?

---

[52] https://www.amazon.com/Do-Not-Consent-Against-Medical-ebook/dp/B08L8JK7FL/

The virus / Tests / Numbers

There is much that is now accepted as "true" about the virus and its origins. We're also fed a daily tally of numbers of cases, hospitalizations, deaths, and vaccines administered. Let's take a look at some of the assumptions we may be making in this area.

The virus came from China

It is almost universally accepted that the virus originally came from the city of Wuhan in China. We don't tend to question this, as we've heard this repeated so often. We're used to hearing reference to "the China Virus", or "WuFlu".

As yet "Patient Zero", the person who was the initial cause of the outbreak, has not been tracked down, despite extensive efforts[53]. Although there are suggestions that authorities in China know the identity of this person, but haven't released details.

The first cases were discovered and reported in early December 2019 in Wuhan, but there are now suggestions that "an unnamed man from China's Hubei province is said to have been the first known case of Covid-19 as early as November 17th 2019"[54].

However, without a definitive "Patient Zero" it really isn't possible to fix the point of origin as Wuhan. Back in March 2020 several Chinese officials put forward the suggestion that U.S. troops could have brought the virus to China from the States, as reported in The Straits Times[55]:

ARTICLE: U.S. military may have brought coronavirus to Wuhan, says China in war of words with U.S.

> A spokesman for China's Foreign Ministry suggested on Thursday (March 12) that the U.S. military might have brought the coronavirus to the Chinese city of Wuhan, which has been hardest hit by the outbreak, doubling down on a war of words with Washington.

---

[53] https://www.bbc.com/future/article/20200221-coronavirus-the-harmful-hunt-for-covid-19s-patient-zero

[54] https://www.mirror.co.uk/news/world-news/one-year-coronavirus-patient-zero-23018740

[55] https://www.straitstimes.com/asia/east-asia/us-military-may-have-brought-coronavirus-to-wuhan-says-china-in-war-of-words-with-us

Perhaps the virus did originate in China, perhaps not. For most of us it is of little real consequence where the virus first infected a human, as it changes nothing about the situation we currently face. However, in the international political arena, where the blame-game of finger pointing and the associated cries for compensation rages on, it is a pretty salient piece of information.

The virus occurred naturally

This was an early bone of contention.

Initial theories pointed to the Huanan Seafood Wholesale Market in Wuhan, one of China's many so-called "wet markets"[56]. The suggestion was that the origin of the virus was a jump from animals to humans through an intermediary host. Most people now accept the story that the two species involved in this jump were bats and pangolins.

However, with the Wuhan Institute of Virology (WIV), a Biosecurity Level 4 (BSL-4) laboratory known to be conducting research on potentially human-infectious coronaviruses, located just a few miles away from the wet market, another potential source of viral outbreak is possible.

Indeed, even before the current pandemic, concerns were expressed about the safety protocols at Chinese virology labs. From the Wikipedia page about WIV[57]:

> Scientists such as U.S. molecular biologist Richard H. Ebright, who had expressed concern of previous escapes of the SARS virus at Chinese laboratories in Beijing and had been troubled by the pace and scale of China's plans for expansion into BSL–4 laboratories, called the Institute a "world-class research institution that does world-class research in virology and immunology" while he noted that the WIV is a world leader in the study of bat coronaviruses.

The quote above comes from the Wikipedia page about the Wuhan Institute of Virology. It is interesting to note that the very next sentence, after stating that scientists had expressed safety concerns about Chinese labs in general, BSL-4 labs in particular, and also pointing out that the WIV was studying bat coronaviruses in particular, is: "The laboratory has nevertheless been the subject of multiple conspiracy theories about the origin of the virus."

---

[56] https://www.businessinsider.com/wuhan-coronavirus-chinese-wet-market-photos-2020-1?IR=T

[57] https://en.wikipedia.org/wiki/Wuhan_Institute_of_Virology

"Multiple conspiracy theories"! That is powerful use of language from a website that purports to be impartial. Because of the negative "tin foil hat", "flat earthers" connotations of the phrase, the feeling this sentence imparts is that any suggestion that the biolab studying bat coronaviruses is involved in any way in the virus spreading to the human population is a ridiculous notion.

Here's more conflicting information about the origins of the virus, from a BBC article[58]:

ARTICLE: Who is 'patient zero' in the coronavirus outbreak?

> However, a study, by Chinese researchers published in the Lancet medical journal, claimed the first person to be diagnosed with Covid-19, was on 1 December 2019 (a lot earlier) and that person had "no contact" with the Huanan Seafood Wholesale Market.
>
> Wu Wenjuan, a senior doctor at Wuhan's Jinyintan Hospital and one of the authors of the study, told the BBC Chinese Service that the patient was an elderly man who suffered from Alzheimer's disease.
>
> "He (the patient) lived four or five buses from the seafood market, and because he was sick he basically didn't go out," Wu Wenjuan said.
>
> She also said that three other people developed symptoms in the following days – two of whom had no exposure to Huanan either.

Here's a different article from The Sun newspaper's website[59], dated 18th Jan 2021, with a different potential "Patient Zero", this time a scientist connected to the WIV.

ARTICLE: VIRUS MYSTERY: Photo emerges 'showing patient zero at Wuhan lab' three years after bosses claimed she left and never to returned

> Huang Yanling, believed to be the world's first coronavirus patient, disappeared 12 months ago amid claims of a cover-up orchestrated by officials in Beijing.

---

[58] https://www.bbc.com/future/article/20200221-coronavirus-the-harmful-hunt-for-covid-19s-patient-zero

[59] https://www.thesun.co.uk/news/13777681/photo-emerges-patient-zero-wuhan-lab-coronavirus/

> At the time, the Wuhan Institute of Virology (WIV) denied online reports the first person to contract the killer virus was based at the top secret site and insisted Huang had left five years earlier never to return.
>
> It [a photo date-stamped 2018 supposedly showing Yanling with a group of other researchers] is believed to have been published on the institute's official website before it was purged of key files related to the outbreak.
>
> "Has WIV been asked to explain why Huang Yanling is present in a 2018 photo if she is said to have left WIV in 2015?"
>
> Since Huang's disappearance, online rumours have circulated in China claiming she died of the virus and was hastily cremated.

Again, any suggestions of this nature tend to be swiftly labelled as "conspiracy theory nonsense" and quietly buried under an on-going avalanche of stories promoting a different narrative.

Who knows what the truth really is?

Back in early 2020, when news of the WIV and its proximity to the wet market first surfaced, anyone who suggested that there may be some connection was ridiculed into silence.

Now there is more open discussion, and on-going investigations as to the real origin of the virus.

If the virus came from a lab, it was an accident

The "evidence" for the laboratory escape of the virus is growing. It is known that scientists at the WIV were involved in what is called "gain of function" studies, where they push viruses to mutate, often in the direction of becoming more virulent, in order to study how best to defend against such viruses if they ever happen to appear naturally in the wild.

That is little like lighting a fire in a tinder-dry forest in order to practice forest fire-fighting techniques. You really hope that the fire doesn't get out of hand.

Of course, it is known that a certain proportion of forest wildfires are started deliberately, sometimes, almost unbelievably, by one of the firefighters from that region, who wants to see some action and be viewed as a hero when they save the day.

A common tactic, used by despotic rulers over the centuries to gain more power and control over a populace, is to create a problem, crank up the levels of fear about this problem until the people are crying out for help, then produce a solution which paints the rulers riding to the rescue in a glow of heroism.

Sound familiar? It's just a thought.

The virus is as dangerous as we're told, and must be stopped at all costs

In the early days of the pandemic it really seemed like we were entering one of the most dangerous periods we had faced globally for a long time. Little was known about the virus.

Estimates of the R-naught, the rate the virus spreads within a population, and projections of potential death rates were terrifying.

One study, based on computer modelling by Imperial College London (ICL) in the UK, and presented by, among others, Neil Ferguson, estimated numbers of deaths in the UK would top 500,000 if no measures to mitigate outcomes were taken. Even with mitigation, Ferguson & Co. claimed, deaths would likely be over 250,000.

Their report was released on March 17th 2020, as detailed by the BBC[60].

ARTICLE: Coronavirus: UK changes course amid death toll fears

> Change course or a quarter of a million people will die in a "catastrophic epidemic" of coronavirus - warnings do not come much starker than that.
>
> The message came from researchers modelling how the disease will spread, how the NHS would be overwhelmed and how many would die.

It was in large part due to this terrifying modelling that the UK government made one of their infamous U-turns, and decided to put the whole nation into strict lockdown.

On 23rd March British Prime Minister Boris Johnson announced people should "stay at home"[61].

---

[60] https://www.bbc.com/news/health-51915302

[61] https://www.telegraph.co.uk/global-health/science-and-disease/terrifying-data-behind-government-coronavirus-lockdown/

Ferguson later tweaked a couple of numbers in the model, and came back almost immediately after the lockdown was announced, with a new estimate of just 20,000, a 90% reduction from his hysterical initial estimates.[62] [63]

Almost a year after the first lockdown began the official UK number of deaths is somewhere between the two estimates, just a touch over 110,000.

We'll look at how these numbers are counted later, but it is interesting to note that there are two ways the UK government categorizes deaths:

- "Deaths within 28 days of positive test"
  110,250 (at 2nd Feb 2021)
- "Deaths with COVID-19 on the death certificate"
  112,660 (at 2nd Feb 2021)

https://coronavirus.data.gov.uk/details/deaths

Ironically, Ferguson was later branded an "arrogant hypocrite", according to a Daily Mail article[64] for encouraging his mistress to break the rules of the lockdown triggered largely because of his own faulty modelling.

ARTICLE: Government scientist Neil Ferguson, 51 - whose death toll projections sparked lockdown - QUITS after admitting he allowed married mistress, 38, to break stay-at-home rules to visit him for trysts

> Professor Neil Ferguson was branded an 'arrogant hypocrite' today for catastrophically 'undermining' the government's position by flouting the strict coronavirus social distancing rules he helped draw up to have secret trysts with his married lover.
>
> The shamed scientist, nicknamed 'Professor Lockdown' because he convinced Boris Johnson to order millions to stay at home, has sensationally quit his Government role on the influential SAGE committee - but his employer Imperial College London is standing by him.

---

[62] https://www.washingtonexaminer.com/news/imperial-college-scientist-who-predicted-500k-coronavirus-deaths-in-uk-revises-to-20k-or-less

[63] https://www.washingtontimes.com/news/2020/mar/26/uk-epidemiologist-radically-lowers-his-predicted-c/

[64] https://www.dailymail.co.uk/news/article-8289921/Scientist-advice-led-lockdown-QUITS-breaking-restrictions-meet-married-lover.html

> Professor Ferguson, 51, asked his mistress Antonia Staats, 38, to travel across London to his home at least twice despite lecturing 66 million in Britain on the need to stay apart to stop the spread of the killer virus.

Seriously, you couldn't make this stuff up, could you?

The current numbers of cases are as reported

During "the first wave" in early 2020 testing for the Sars-CoV-2 virus was very limited. The reagents needed to make the PCR (Polymerase Chain Reaction) test kits were in limited supply. In the UK you had to practically be on death's doorstep before you could get tested.

A year later there are many test kits available from different manufacturers and testing is done in huge numbers. In the UK, for example, on 3rd February 2021, over 800,000 tests were done, resulting in almost 20,000 new "cases".[65]

Over the past months these "cases" have been one of the main drivers for the continued lockdowns and restrictions upon our freedoms. They also support the "everyone needs to be vaccinated as soon as humanly possible" narrative.

But it is important to realise that not all of these "cases" are actually cases by medical definition, but are merely positive test results. And there is also much doubt about the accuracy of the tests too... which we'll come to shortly.

From Wikipedia's "Clinical case definition page"[66]:

> "In epidemiology, a clinical case definition, a clinical definition, or simply a case definition lists the clinical criteria by which public health professionals determine whether a person's illness is included as a case in an outbreak investigation."

Many people who receive a positive test result have no symptoms, don't feel ill, and are completely unaware that they are "infected". It is very hard to say that they have an "illness", as per the definition above.

They perhaps have had to have a test because of requirements where they work, or because they had plans to travel. If they hadn't had to be tested, they may have never known that they were "positive".

---

[65] https://coronavirus.data.gov.uk/details/cases

[66] https://en.wikipedia.org/wiki/Clinical_case_definition

If you haven't turned up at your doctor's office, or headed for the hospital, you're not really a case, are you?

The PCR tests are reliable and accurate

It has been known for quite some time that PCR tests often return "false positives". This happens because of the way the test works. The sample taken has to be multiplied many many times to create enough material for a test to analyse. Each multiplication, or replication, doubles the sample size, and is called a "cycle".

The less cycles required to find measurable virus particles mean there is a higher viral load in the initial sample. The point at which the virus can be found is called the cycle threshold (Ct).

Running tests at high cycle thresholds can produce positive results from tiny particles of dead virus in the original sample, perhaps from a previous infection. This means that a person who is no longer infected, and has fought off the virus, perhaps without realizing they ever had it, can get a positive result and be diagnosed as a "new case".

This December 18th 2020 article[67] does a much better job of explaining all this than I can, and directly quotes CDC (U.S. Centers for Disease Control and Prevention) guidelines on cycle thresholds.

ARTICLE: WHO (finally) admits PCR tests create false positives:

From the article:

> This new WHO memo states that using a high CT value to test for the presence of SARS-CoV-2 will result in false-positive results.
>
> To quote their own words [our emphasis]:
>
> > "Users of RT-PCR reagents should read the IFU carefully to determine if manual adjustment of the PCR positivity threshold is necessary to account for any background noise which **may lead to a specimen with a high cycle threshold (Ct) value result being interpreted as a positive result**."
>
> They go on to explain [again, our emphasis]:

---

[67] https://off-guardian.org/2020/12/18/who-finally-admits-pcr-tests-create-false-positives/

> "The design principle of RT-PCR means that for patients with high levels of circulating virus (viral load), relatively few cycles will be needed to detect virus and so the Ct value will be low. Conversely, when specimens return a high Ct value, it means that many cycles were required to detect virus. **In some circumstances, the distinction between background noise and actual presence of the target virus is difficult to ascertain.**"

Of course, none of this is news to anyone who has been paying attention.

Also from the article:

> Dr Kary Mullis, who won the Nobel Prize for inventing the PCR process, was clear that it wasn't meant as a diagnostic tool, saying:
>
> > "with PCR, if you do it well, you can find almost anything in anybody."

And finally:

> Even Dr Anthony Fauci has publicly admitted that a cycle threshold over 35 is going to be detecting "dead nucleotides", not a living virus.
>
> Despite all this, it is known that many labs around the world have been using PCR tests with CT values over 35, even into the low 40s.

Now, you have to wonder, don't you, why they might want case numbers to be artificially inflated by running tests way above the recommended threshold for effective diagnosis?

Here's another interesting article from September 29th 2020[68]:

ARTICLE: Coronavirus Cases Plummet When PCR Tests Are Adjusted:

From the article:

> In three sets of testing data that include cycle thresholds compiled by officials in Massachusetts, New York and Nevada, up to 90 percent of people testing positive carried barely any virus, a review by The New York Times found.

[68] https://thevaccinereaction.org/2020/09/coronavirus-cases-plummet-when-pcr-tests-are-adjusted/

And:

> Any test with a cycle threshold (CT) above 35 is too sensitive, says Juliet Morrison, PhD, a virologist at the University of California, Riverside. "I'm shocked that people would think that 40 [cycles] could represent a positive." A more reasonable cutoff would be 30 to 35, she added. Dr. Mina said he would set the figure at 30, or even less. Those changes would mean the amount of genetic material in a patient's sample would have to be 100-fold to 1,000-fold that of the current standard for the test to return a positive result worth acting on.
>
> The CDC's own calculations suggest that it is extremely difficult to detect any live virus in a sample above a threshold of 33 cycles.

All comments in the above article contain reference links to original source materials.

The numbers of deaths are as reported

In the UK, as previously mentioned, deaths are either counted as "Deaths within 28 days of positive test", or as "Deaths with COVID-19 on the death certificate"

Both numbers seem to produce similar daily results.

Neither of these numbers actually tells us how many people died from COVID-19, as this is very different from a death that occurs within 28 days of a positive test.

More to the point, these numbers don't tell us how many people died from COVID-19 alone, and had no other underlying health problems. Surely that would be a more accurate measure of how deadly the disease is?

By this bizarre method of classification, someone who dies in a motorcycle accident within 4 weeks of a positive test can be counted as a "COVID death". A heart attack days or weeks after a positive test can be added to the mounting COVID death tally.

It's almost as ridiculous as asking how many people ate cheesecake in the previous month, and then listing cheesecake as the cause of death for anyone unfortunate enough to pass on within the arbitrarily allotted timeframe.

There is no prophylaxis or treatment option

Oh dear! This particular assumption, or choosing to believe this part of the story we're being told, brings us to the entrance to a rather deep rabbit warren of conjecture, claims and counter-claims, lies, censorship, as well as some high-level political manouvering and back-stabbing.

Few people will be unaware of the controversy that surrounded the use of Hydroxychloroquine as a early treatment for coronavirus cases. The drug very quickly shifted from being considered a very safe prophylaxis (preventative) for malaria to becoming a dangerous drug with serious potential to produce heart arrhythmia.

When President Trump suggested this cheap, off-patent (any company can produce it as nobody owns a patent for it) medicine was a potential "game changer" he was mocked and ridiculed in the media.

And anyone who tried to discuss the matter, even qualified doctors who were having great success using HCQ as a treatment, were silenced and censored on social media.

This 28th January 2021 article on TheGatewayPundit website[69] refers to a posting in October from a Facebook user in France which Facebook moderators removed as it contravened their "misinformation and imminent harm rule".

Article: After 440,000 Americans are Dead – Facebook and American Journal of Medicine Admit Their Stand on HCQ was Wrong – These People Should be Prosecuted!

> Today that number [deaths in the USA] is at 440,000.
>
> We now know that that number could have been lowered significantly if HCQ use would have been promoted in the US!

Here's what the Oversight Board said as they overturned, in January 2021, Facebook's decision to remove the post[70]:

> In October 2020, a user posted a video and accompanying text in French in a public Facebook group related to COVID-19. The post alleged a scandal at the Agence Nationale de Sécurité du Médicament (the French agency responsible for regulating health products), which refused to authorise hydroxychloroquine combined with azithromycin for use against COVID-19, but

---

[69] https://www.thegatewaypundit.com/2021/01/440000-americans-dead-facebook-american-journal-medicine-admit-stand-hcq-wrong-people-prosecuted/

[70] https://oversightboard.com/news/325131635492891-oversight-board-overturns-facebook-decision-case-2020-006-fb-fbr/

> authorised and promoted remdesivir. The user criticised the lack of a health strategy in France and stated that "[Didier] Raoult's cure" is being used elsewhere to save lives. The user's post also questioned what society had to lose by allowing doctors to prescribe in an emergency a "harmless drug" when the first symptoms of COVID-19 appear.
>
> Facebook removed the content for violating its misinformation and imminent harm rule, which is part of its violence and incitement Community Standard, finding the post contributed to the risk of imminent physical harm during a global pandemic. Facebook explained that it removed the post as it contained claims that a cure for COVID-19 exists. The company concluded that this could lead people to ignore health guidance or attempt to self-medicate.

Eight months after Donald Trump's "game changer" ponderings were mocked, as more and more research seems to indicate very positive results when HCQ is used as early treatment, a study posted in the American Journal of Medicine[71] in January 2021 found that early treatment of coronavirus patients with hydroxychloroquine could lower the mortality rate for the disease.

We'll discuss HCQ along with another cheap, off-patent medicine showing very positive results when we discuss inoculations, and particularly the Emergency Use Authorizations which allow early use of these experimental vaccines.

---

[71] https://www.amjmed.com/article/S0002-9343(20)30673-2/fulltext

Lockdowns / The economy

Lockdowns are inevitably causing significant harm, not just to the economy, but to our personal wellbeing. Depending on rules where you live, you may be restricted in movement, unable to visit loved ones, unable to operate your business, or enjoy many of the freedoms we took for granted just one year ago. What assumptions are being made?

Lockdowns are necessary to stop our health systems being overwhelmed

Before the coronavirus pandemic struck, lockdowns as we know them today had never been used as a mitigation strategy for any viral outbreak.

The strategy outlined by the WHO and other bodies has always been to quarantine the infected, protect the most vunerable, and let others get on pretty much as normal.

Why then did China initiate such a strict lockdown, and why have western nations on the whole followed suit?

As discussed in the previous section, computer modelling produced some terrifying numbers, and lockdowns followed quickly afterwards. Was this wise mitigation, and are we benefitting later from the prompt actions of our leaders? Or was it a knee-jerk reaction caused by fear and panic?

Alex Berenson, in his book "Unreported Truths About Covid-19 and Lockdowns"[72], (which was originally banned by Amazon until Elon Musk tweeted about it[73]) suggests the answer is simple:

> The most likely explanation is the simplest. Faced with a risk of hundreds of thousands or millions of deaths, the public health experts who for decades had counseled patience and caution flinched. They found they could not live with acknowledging how little control they or any of us had over the spread of an easily transmissible respiratory virus. They had to do something – even if they had been warning for decades that what they were about to do would not work and might have terrible secondary consequences.

---

[72] https://www.amazon.com/Unreported-Truths-About-Covid-19-Lockdowns-ebook/dp/B08QND25GL/

[73] https://www.cnbc.com/2020/06/04/elon-musk-calls-for-amazon-split-after-alex-berenson-claims-censorship.html

Almost a year later lockdowns are back, as "cases" increase, and yet we still have no real proof that lockdowns actually achieve anything.

In Sweden, for example, where during the first wave there was no lockdown at all, numbers of hospitalizations and numbers of deaths were very similar to neighbouring Nordic countries who implemented strict lockdowns.

We're told lockdowns are necessary for our safety, and we generally just accept it, despite the horrendous costs personally in both financial terms and our mental wellbeing.

We must all make sacrifices to stop the virus

It seems that the only deaths that count anymore are COVID deaths. COVID deaths must be prevented at all costs.

Lockdowns have meant many elective surgeries have been cancelled. Scans and diagnoses for cancer have been delayed.

People have been locked in their homes for weeks, sometimes months on end. The emotional toll is terrible. Many have seen their businesses shuttered, probably never to re-open in some cases. The personal financial devastation is immeasurable. Alcohol and drug abuse has increased, as has domestic violence. Suicide rates are on the rise.

But none of this seems to matter. COVID must be stopped, and mitigation measures will continue until everybody has been vaccinated.

The economy will "bounce back" in a v-shaped recovery

One of the greatest casualties of the lockdowns is going to be the economy. In many countries the awful toll this is going to have on businesses and jobs is currently hidden by furlough payments, loan schemes and welfare benefit increases.

How long can governments go on creating currency out of thin air to pay people to stay at home watching Netflix?

When the stimulus payments and furloughs eventually wind down the terrible consequences of lockdowns will finally be revealed.

An article on MarketWatch.com, last updated on 10th February 2021[74] explains how "some 11.4 million Americans will be cut off from receiving

---

[74] https://www.marketwatch.com/story/over-11-million-americans-face-an-unemployment-cliff-if-lawmakers-dont-extend-covid-19-relief-programs-11612281710

unemployment benefits between March 14 and April 11" unless further government assistance is agreed upon.

ARTICLE: Over 11 million Americans face an unemployment cliff if lawmakers don't extend COVID-19 relief programs:

> It's likely that jobless Americans will continue to receive enhanced unemployment given that it's included in President Joe Biden's $1.9-trillion stimulus package proposal, as well as a counter stimulus proposal supported by at least 10 Republican lawmakers.
>
> Biden's package calls for increasing the enhanced benefits to $400 per week through September.

Many businesses forced to close their doors because of mandated restrictions are thought to have gone out of business completely, never to reopen again, according to this CNN article[75].

ARTICLE: Yikes! Yelp says 60% of restaurant Covid-19 closures are permanent:

> "The restaurant industry now reflects the highest total business closures, recently surpassing retail," Yelp says.
>
> Many have tried to adapt with online ordering, curbside pickup and home delivery.
>
> As of July 10, Yelp found 26,160 total restaurant closures, an increase of 2,179 since June 15.
>
> Of all the closed restaurants in July, 15,770 have permanently closed (60%), accounting for 2,956 more permanent closures, Yelp says. That's a 23% increase since June 15.

Will the economy bounce back in the fabled "v-shaped recovery"? A lot of people have been saving the extra bounty governments have bestowed upon them through the crisis, and there are some suggestions that a pent-up demand to consume, to travel, to spend will jolt the economy back to life.

But due to massive money printing, there is also the potential for this spending binge, if it does actually happen, to result in rampant price inflation.

---

[75] https://edition.cnn.com/2020/07/25/business/restaurants-reopen-coronavirus-shutdown-trnd/index.html

What do you think? Are we going back to "business as usual" as soon as the vaccine roll-out is finished? Does the economy just need a quick jolt, and we're off and running again?

You don't have to look very far to find an army of credible economists suggesting we may be looking at a depression worse than the 1930s Great Depression, and that we have a "lost decade" ahead of us.

Vaccines / Outcomes

Finally, let's take a look at assumptions built in to the story we're being told about the vaccine roll-out.

The vaccines are necessary

In order to accept what we're told about the vaccines – that they are necessary, safe and effective – we are required to put a lot of faith in the companies who have rushed through these treatments in record time.

Vaccines are being rolled out across the globe on an Emergency Use basis, on the strength of research done by the vaccine companies themselves.

NOTE: we'll take a closer look at Emergency Use Authorization (EUA) in Part 5, when we dive deeper into vaccines.

Phase 3 trials hastily completed on limited numbers of research subjects "prove", according to the manufacturers, that the vaccines are safe, and are effective, with some claiming more than 90% efficacy.

By the very nature of the timeline involved any safety and efficacy results can only be judged in the short term. How the vaccines might work (or not work) in the medium term, or in the long term is completely unknown at this point.

Without long term studies monitored by independent scientists, accepting results from the big pharma companies without asking any questions at all is a little like believing the tobacco companies own research, from short term, hastily completed studies, when they initially claimed their products caused no harm.

If you were desperate for a smoke, it was easy to ignore the concerned little voice in the back of your mind which wondered if the tobacco company was telling the truth, just as if you're desperate now for lockdowns to be over and life to return to normal, it is easy to believe that the vaccine will provide the quick fix you desire so badly.

The vaccines are safe

The U.S. Department of Health and Human Services (HHS) provide a website where vaccine adverse events can be reported, called the Vaccine Adverse Event Reporting System (VAERS)[76].

---

[76] https://vaers.hhs.gov/index.html

It takes a while to figure out how to filter and use the data available, but there is a wealth of information on reactions to vaccines.

Filtering for COVID-19 vaccines only (10th February 2021), and for the "adverse reaction event" of "death" produces a surprising total of 501 "events". 271 of those events are related to the Pfizer/BioNTech vaccine, 228 to the Moderna vaccine, and 2 deaths related to "unknown manufacturer".

Now, I'm not a statistician, so haven't studied these figures in depth, but it is easy for the layman researcher to see that the bulk of these deaths have occurred in higher age groups. Many events involve other complications, patients who are taking other drugs, or who have other health issues.

In fact, when you look at the detailed information on each reported event, the website states: "Submitting a report to VAERS does not mean that healthcare personnel or the vaccine caused or contributed to the adverse event (possible side effect)."

So it isn't possible to directly attribute a particular death directly to a vaccination, but there are more than enough cases to raise doubts.

Here, for example, VAERS ID: 0994913-1 details a 48 year old female, given the Moderna vaccine on 30th January 2021, who died two days later. The Adverse Event Description reads: "patient passed away 2 days after vaccine. patient had temperature, nausea, and vomiting after vaccine."

There are plenty of other similar "events" reported. Surely enough to call into question possible safety implications, particularly if you are older, have underlying health issues, or are taking other drugs?

Although, of course, you'll hear very little about the 12,000+ COVID-19 adverse events reported to date in the mainstream media, as they seem determined to keep pushing the "vaccines are safe" message at all costs.

Begin your search here:
https://wonder.cdc.gov/vaers.html

Adverse events update 18th February 2021

I just found this enlightening article[77] on VaccineImpact.com, dated 13th February 2021, which gives more details on reports of deaths after COVID

[77] https://vaccineimpact.com/2021/cdc-witholding-information-1170-dead-following-covid-injections-almost-twice-as-many-deaths-as-found-in-vaers/

vaccinations, and has a link to a great source of easy-to-understand data pulled from the VAERS database.

ARTICLE: CDC WITHOLDING INFORMATION! 1,170 DEAD Following COVID Injections: Almost Twice as Many Deaths as Found in VAERS

> Yesterday we reported that the CDC had done another data dump into the VAERS (Vaccine Adverse Event Reporting System) database, showing that through February 4, 2021, there were 12,697 recorded adverse events, including 653 deaths following injections of the experimental COVID mRNA shots by Pfizer and Moderna.
>
> After publishing this article, a Health Impact News subscriber sent me a link to a page on the CDC website where they are reporting that as of February 11, 2021, VAERS received 1,170 reports of death among people who received a COVID-19 vaccine.

The writer has a theory about the big discrepancy in numbers:

> For the past few weeks, the CDC has been slowly updating the VAERS database with data dumps on Friday, just before the weekend and the beginning of the slow news cycle that usually picks up again on Mondays.
>
> On Friday, January 29th, their VAERS data reported 329 deaths from people receiving one of the experimental COVID mRNA injections.
>
> The following Friday, February 5, 2021, their VAERS data reported 501 deaths. An increase of 172 deaths.
>
> Yesterday, February 12, 2021, the CDC VAERS data reported 653 deaths. An increase of 152 deaths.
>
> That still leaves 517 deaths unaccounted for in the VAERS database related to the COVID injections.
>
> Why is the CDC withholding this information?

The article contains a link to a page on the CDC website which, although last time I visited (2 days ago on 16th February) did indeed say there had been 1,170 deaths reported after a vaccination, today (18th February) it now reads:

> Over 52 million doses of COVID-19 vaccines were administered in the United States from December 14, 2020, through February

> 14, 2021. During this time, VAERS received 934 reports of death (0.0018%) among people who received a COVID-19 vaccine.

It must have been a miscount a couple of days ago!?! Or did 236 reports go into the shredder?

I found it interesting to note that the CDC had a bulletpoint list of things they feel we need to know:

> What you need to know:
>
> - COVID-19 vaccines are safe and effective.
> - Millions of people in the United States have received COVID-19 vaccines, and these vaccines will undergo the most intensive safety monitoring in U.S. history.
> - CDC recommends you get a COVID-19 vaccine as soon as you are eligible.

So, wait a minute... bulletpoint 1 states that the vaccines are safe and effective and in point 3 we're urged to get one as soon as humanly possible. Meanwhile, point 2 assures us that "these vaccines **will** undergo the most intensive safety monitoring". [emphasis added]

Will? I'd rather wait until a significant amount of safety monitoring **has been** done.

The VaccineImpact article also links to this great resource, which pulls data directly from the VAERS database, but displays it in a much easier to understand format:
https://medalerts.org/vaersdb/findfield.php?TABLE=ON&GROUP1=AGE&EVENTS=ON&ESORT=VAX-DATE&VAX=COVID19&DIED=Yes

The vaccines are effective

Due to the rushed Emergency Use Authorization for the newly created vaccines, many questions about their efficacy still remain unanswered.

- How long until a vaccine creates immunity?
- How long does immunity last?
- Will the vaccine work for everyone?
- What level of immunity does a single dose achieve?
- Will new variants be covered by a vaccine?
- Will we need booster shots each year?
- What if the recipient has already had COVID-19?

If you answer any of the above questions with the response, "We just don't know" then you'd be getting close to the answers you'll find to these questions from the producers of these treatments.

As there have been no medium-term or long-term results yet, we're still firmly in the land of guesswork and hope.

Vaccination will help us reach herd immunity

What percentage of the population need to be vaccinated to achieve herd immunity?

"We just don't know!"

Anthony Fauci admitted to altering his "guidance" several times, as reported in this FoxNews article[78]:

ARTICLE: Fauci shifts herd immunity goalposts, now says as much as 90% may be needed to halt coronavirus

> Fauci indicated that he based his shifting statements on public polling on the popularity of coronavirus vaccines.
>
> "When polls said only about half of all Americans would take a vaccine, I was saying herd immunity would take 70 to 75 percent," Fauci said. "Then, when newer surveys said 60 percent or more would take it, I thought, 'I can nudge this up a bit,' so I went to 80, 85."
>
> He continued: "We really don't know what the real number is. I think the real range is somewhere between 70 to 90 percent. But, I'm not going to say 90 percent."

So, not so much "following the science", but more "Let's see what we can get away with based on the polling results".

We will be able to return to some semblance of normality if we all do what we're told

Finally, if you're going to go along unquestioningly with the entire narrative, you have to belive, or at least hope, that once we're all vaccinated, things will go back to normal, or something like normal.

I feel the same desire as I imagine you do to be done with all of this, to go back to the world we knew and loved as it was in January 2020.

---

[78] https://www.foxnews.com/politics/fauci-shift-herd-immunity-90-percent

What do you miss the most? Shopping, travel, concerts, eating out, the pub, movies, the theatre, going to the gym, visiting friends and family?

We've lost so much, and after a year of challenges and changes, it is so easy to grasp at straws. The promise of a vaccine quick fix to all of this is so appealing, so it is easy to simply go along without thinking too much, hoping all will be resolved within a couple of months.

However, once vaccinated, we're now told, we'll still have to wear masks, practice social distancing and abide by lockdown rules or curfew regulations. All this because you might still be infectious, even if you aren't symptomatic, so you're still going to have to wait quite some time before all restrictions are lifted.

It seems likely that lockdowns will be on-again off-again at least until the vaccine roll-out is almost complete.

In the meantime we're already hearing of "new variant" strains of the virus, and even tougher restrictive measures are being discussed. Will the vaccine be effective against these mutations, or will we need booster shots? Maybe, like flu vaccines, we'll need a new one every year.

Perhaps as new variants emerge we'll be locked down again until we're all re-immunised!

PART 4: THE NARRATIVE WE CHOOSE

"Every record has been destroyed or falsified, every book rewritten, every picture has been repainted, every statue and street building has been renamed, every date has been altered. And the process is continuing day by day and minute by minute. History has stopped. Nothing exists except an endless present in which the Party is always right."

George Orwell

1984

I want to believe

Cult 90s TV series "The X-Files"[79] carried the tagline "I want to believe".

Fox Mulder, maverick FBI agent tasked with studying the strange, unusual, mysterious cases that nobody else wanted to investigate, often found himself siding with the conspiracy theorists. His partner, Dana Scully, provided some balance, combining a deep scepticism with a rigorous scientific approach.

The larger story arc which continued through all the series, and in a couple of movies too, involved a massive government cover-up of the discovery of alien technology, and the subsequent use of that technology for evil intent.

"I want to believe" was the phrase on a poster, occasionally seen in an episode, on Fox Mulder's basement office wall. The words appeared below an image of a UFO. Fox was clearly deeply invested in believing in the plot he was trying to uncover.

The X-Files was a huge success, perhaps partly due to the fact that we all enjoy an occasional visit to the deep rabbit hole of conspiracy theories.

But perhaps we can take the phrase "I want to believe", and turn it on its head in regard to our current situation.

Instead of using it to indicate a desire to embrace all of the darkest ideas of evil goings-on behind the scenes, we can acknowledge that the world would be a better place if we really could believe the stories we are told.

Our recent past has been filled with challenges, changes, loss of freedoms, and fear. The easiest and most comforting option is to take all we're told at face value, and go along for the ride.

In February and March I did believe. I thought, based on what I read and heard, that we were facing a tidal wave of disease and death. I believed the news reports, I understood how exponential growth hides the numbers until they explode off the chart. I saw the haggard doctors in Italy. I saw the reasoning which led to the first lockdown in the UK, because it was necessary to "flatten the curve". I was an early adopter of mask use. I believed.

But little by little, over the months, things just haven't seemed to add up. I began to question what was going on as governments made decisions, then hasty U-turns, as masks weren't essential, then suddenly were mandated, as lockdowns destroyed businesses, lives and the economy.

---

[79] https://www.imdb.com/title/tt0106179/

I was amazed to see what appeared to be very obvious censorship as any discussion of Hydroxychloroquine was sidelined and ridiculed, and qualified doctors were de-platformed for expressing an opinion which differed from that constantly being pushed in the media.

But it wasn't until the surprise "Hey Presto!" vaccine announcements in early December, months if not years ahead of any predicted timeline, that I really sat up and took any notice.

The final straw that broke the camel's back for me was the hasty approval for emergency use, and the enormous effort to get needles into arms before the ink on the pharma company research papers had had time to dry.

I sincerely hope that I am wrong to be so sceptical.

I hope that we are being told the truth. I hope that the people making decisions for us, enforcing new rules and regulations, and encouraging us to be vaccinated as soon as possible do indeed have our best interests at heart.

I hope that by rolling out a vaccine we find a way to halt the progress of this pandemic, and that our lives will return to normal.

But I don't think I can choose to believe this simplistic narrative any longer.

Who can you trust?

One of the biggest challenges we face in today's modern, connected world, is finding reputable, impartial, accurate and trustworthy sources of news. The problem we have isn't a lack of choice. We are overloaded with information, but as we've seen, doubt is easily cast upon the impartial and unbiased nature of many of these sources.

Much of the information we can access is very contradictory. One report will offer one side of a topic, a different story will offer a polar opposite view. One need look no further than political discussion in many countries to see how divided opinion can become. Each side of the political divide will have their own preferred sources of "facts", and ultimately their own version of the "truth". When the rift between two sets of beliefs is wide enough, there is no way to come to any sort of agreement, and bitter rivalries become self-reinforcing.

When you really think about it, we have no way at all of evaluating the veracity of anything we are told. We can merely consider the source, and do the best we can to build our own beliefs about how the world around us operates.

In simpler times this wasn't such a big problem. Go back a couple of centuries and generally our lives were lived on much smaller stages. As a part of the general population, all we really needed to know about was how things worked in our local area, who could be trusted among the people we mixed with on a daily basis, and perhaps what our local rulers were planning, and what they required from us.

Over the course of the previous century the local newspaper could provide just about all the information we needed, and it was quite possible that you might even know the local publisher, and be able to form an opinion on his trustworthiness and his biases.

Today's world is much more global, and issues on the other side of the world can soon impact our lives in ways we couldn't possibly imagine, as we've seen recently. Trade, conflicts, environmental issues and health crises all play out on an international scale, and we are all involved.

Our need to know has expanded at the same time as our ability to find the real truth has diminished.

Throughout this book I have tried as best I can to avoid presenting anything as "factual", or as "the truth". The problem is that I just don't know what is true, and what is fake. None of us, if we're honest, has any real ability to assess how "truthful" anything we read or hear actually is.

As an example, let's imagine a newspaper, or its website, says there were 2,000 more COVID deaths today. Is that deaths "from COVID", or "deaths within 28 days of a positive test"? Did those who died have any other underlying health issues? What were the age ranges of those who died? Where did the newspaper get this number? From a government talking head at a news conference? How do we know the information he has is accurate? Where did he get the number from? How are the numbers collected on a daily basis from hundreds of hospitals and nursing homes around the country, as well as other deaths that happen within the general populace? How many levels of bureaucracy do these numbers pass through before some statistician collates them and hands them up the chain of managers, until the government spokesman issues his statement?

Even something as simple as tallying up numbers can be called into question. But what about when a pharma company claims that its hot-off-the-press new high-tech experimental vaccine is safe? How do we assess how true that statement is?

We also need to be mindful to be equally sceptical when someone on the other side of the fence claims they have the facts, and we should try to question their claims in the same way.

When someone claims "FACT: They're going to crash the world economy, and we're all going to be slaves controlled by a manipulated digital currency by this time next year!" it is time to ask some questions.

Who are "they"? How are they going to achieve this? What is the motive? What sources are you basing this idea on? What makes you think this is true?

The important thing to realise is that most people's "facts" are merely opinions, and I'd urge a greater degree of scepticism about anything anyone claims is "the truth", whichever side of the narrative they stand on.

Usually someone who claims to know "the truth" has made up their mind, and invested everything into their belief system, and will most likely be unable to alter their ideas, even if presented with new information that conflicts with their current beliefs.

All we can do is try to be as balanced as possible in the sources we refer to, try to put all the information together into an opinion that fits with our understanding of what is going on around us, and then not make the mistake of being so arrogant as to try to force this opinion upon others as "fact".

The truth is a slippery concept, and ultimately the only opinion that really matters is your own. Trust yourself, rather than following any particular narrative. Question, examine and think, and always be prepared to change your opinion in the light of new information

An alternate reality

Maybe then, we're not being told "the truth, the whole truth, and nothing but the truth"? Perhaps there are other things going on that are not clear to us.

As we've discovered, it's impossible to know what the real truth might be, but it is possible to connect some of the dots we can see, and come to a different conclusion to the one which is fed to us as an easy-to-accept simple narrative.

Let's begin with an easy step...

Do you believe the big pharmaceutical companies have our best interests at heart?

Are they motivated to keep us fit and healthy? Does their business model rely upon providing us with the best medications possible? Is their goal to heal us, ensuring we never have to come back for more medicine?

Are they motivated by altruistic goals, and are the billions of dollars of profit they make every year simply just a fortunate outcome from the products they sell?

Or are they driven, like many other businesses, by profit margins, share price valuations, and the desire to build a large base of repeat customers?

Let's, for the sake of this discussion, assume that profit is a big part of the major drug companies' motivation in the competitive marketplace in which they operate.

Next, is it within the realms of possibility that with billions of dollars of past profits, and the prospect of billions more to come, they might want to exert some influence in the media, and in the corridors of power? That kind of money buys a lot of influence, and supports a lot of media empires with lucrative advertising deals.

So with a pandemic running out of control, is it possible to believe that pharma giants see the potential profits in finding a vaccine as quickly as possible, getting it approved for use in record time, and having governments and the media on board to persuade the whole world to roll up their sleeves and get in line?

Not too farfetched, is it?

Let's take the next little step...

Could it be possible that scientists, while working on "gain of function" mutations in bat coronaviruses, so that they could start to develop potential vaccines should such a virus ever develop naturally in the wild, had a bit of a lab accident, allowing the virus to escape?

The first response would probably be to try to cover up the accident.

But once the cat (or bat) is out of the bag, the next course of action would be to find a possible natural source to blame for the new virus. Perhaps something like a pangolin in a wet market just down the road? And then ridicule any suggestion that the lab had anything to do with it.

It's just a coincidence that the lab is only up the road, and is studying forced mutations in bat coronaviruses. To suggest otherwise is obviously a ridiculous conspiracy theory.

Once the virus spreads internationally the same people who funded the gain of function research would be frantically working on a vaccine, because every cloud has a silver lining. Unless they were almost at the point of having a vaccine ready. In which case they'd be able to announce the "development" of a new vaccine in record time. Maybe around 8 or 9 months might be a believable time period to wait before announcing the good news.

STOP THE PRESS !!

A study published by Dr. Steven Quay on 29th January 2021 concludes that there is a "99.8% probability SARS-CoV-2 came from a laboratory." I like the title of the article which I found on TheNationalPulse.com[80], which reads:

CLAIM: Analysis Proves COVID Is Lab-Made Virus

The analysis doesn't "prove" anything, and the doctor only claims a certain (very high) percentage of probability, therefore it is refreshing to see a title which states this is a claim, not a fact. The author is wisely reserving judgement.

From the TheNationalPulse article:

> The author, Dr. Steven Quay, has 360+ published medical studies and has been cited over 10,000 times, placing him in the top one percent of scientists worldwide.

And quoting Dr. Quay directly:

---

[80] https://thenationalpulse.com/breaking/covid-made-in-lab/

> "By taking only publicly available, scientific evidence about SARS-CoV-2 and using highly conservative estimates in my analysis, I nonetheless conclude that it is beyond a reasonable doubt that SARS-CoV-2 escaped from a laboratory."

Dr. Quay's video intro to his paper can be seen here. It's on YouTube, so I suggest you watch it before it gets taken down for "spreading misinformation" or "endangering public health" or something else equally vague:
https://www.youtube.com/watch?v=ATUtjvgT8iI

Dr. Quay's paper is 193 pages long. I have to be honest, I haven't read it all. But if you wish to do so it can be downloaded here:
https://zenodo.org/record/4477081#.YBVzC2Ruc-Q

I'll just quote this one section from page 3:

> The Chinese government, WHO, media, and many academic virologists have stated with strong conviction that the coronavirus came from nature, either directly from bats or indirectly from bats through another species. Transmission of a virus from animals to humans is called a zoonosis.
>
> A small but growing number of scientists have considered another hypothesis: that an ancestral bat coronavirus was collected in the wild, genetically manipulated in a laboratory to make it more infectious, training it to infect human cells, and ultimately released, **probably by accident**, in Wuhan, China.
>
> **For most of 2020 this hypothesis was considered a crackpot idea**, but in the last few weeks, more media attention has been given to the possibility that the Wuhan Institute of Virology, located near the Wuhan city center and with a population of over 11 million inhabitants, may have been the source of the field specimen collection effort, laboratory genetic manipulation, and subsequent leak.
>
> On January 15, 2021, the U.S. Department of State issued a statement requesting the WHO investigation of the origin of COVID-19 include specific assertions related to a laboratory origin of the pandemic. [emphasis added]

Another small step...

In late 2019 an international group ran a pandemic simulation exercise to assess global preparedness for a potential viral outbreak. It was called Event 201. From the World Economic Forum (more about WEF later) website[81]:

> The Johns Hopkins Center for Health Security in partnership with the World Economic Forum and the Bill & Melinda Gates Foundation will host Event 201: a high-level simulation exercise for pandemic preparedness and response, in New York, USA, on Friday 18 October (2019)

Wow. Just two months before the first cases of what would become known as COVID-19 were found in Wuhan. Just a coincidence of course, anything else would be... yes, you've guessed it... a conspiracy theory. The front page of the Event 201 website now carries a link to a comment pointing out that the exercise was "not a prediction".[82]

Even more coincidentally, the scenario imagined a new coronavirus, initially found in animals (pigs) before making the jump to humans. "Infected people got a respiratory illness with symptoms ranging from mild flu-like signs to severe pneumonia. The sickest required intensive care and many died."

You can watch video highlights of the event here:
https://www.youtube.com/watch?v=AoLw-Q8X174

The blurb at the start of the video states: "On average the WHO responds to 200 epidemic events each year. We need to prepare for the event that becomes a pandemic."

They didn't leave much time for preparation.

So here's our next small step

Did someone high up in a pharma company with some promising vaccine candidates coming up for trial wonder how much profit was there to be made by having something like Event 201 become a reality?

Perhaps a virus escaping from a Bio Security Level 4 wasn't really an accident at all?

Is that a believable possibility?

---

81 https://www.weforum.org/press/2019/10/live-simulation-exercise-to-prepare-public-and-private-leaders-for-pandemic-response

82 https://www.centerforhealthsecurity.org/event201/

Here's another small step...

Perhaps the pharma companies weren't involved in the manufacture or the release of the virus at all, and are just profiteering now from what are, for them, a happy series of coincidental events.

As Seneca once said, "Luck is what happens when preparation meets opportunity."

So how about this as a possibility? The virus never came from that lab at all, but was released in that vicinity, so that obvious conclusions would be easy to draw.

Which fading world superpower might be sufficiently motivated to release a virus close to a Chinese BSL-4 lab, and then act outraged, but be secretly delighted when China's rising star begins to dim again?

I wonder...

A magical misdirection

What if this isn't just about managing a viral outbreak?

Just as a magician uses misdirection to focus the audience's attention away from the secret of the illusion, so too could the pandemic be used to refocus our attention away from other events which we're not supposed to notice.

With the world economy in 2019 taking on the appearance of a giant bubble in search of a pin, perhaps the pandemic provides the perfect cover for a disastrous financial crisis.

In January 2020 U.S. debt was just a touch over $23 trillion. A year later current U.S. national debt stands at just under $28 trillion[83]. By the time this book goes to print, if the current proposal for a further $1.9 trillion of spending is approved, debt will possibly top $30 trillion.

This increase in debt to the tune of trillions of dollars has allowed the government to send out occasional "stimulus checks" to most citizens as businesses remained shuttered, while simultaneously somehow helping the stock market attain new highs after its initial stumble in March 2020.

The European Central Bank and the Bank Of England have been similarly magnanimous in the creation out of thin air of ridiculous amounts of currency, in an effort to keep all the plates spinning.

---

[83] https://usdebtclock.org/

Now, however, instead of governments and central banks being blamed for their reckless financial engineering, massive currency creation, and market manipulation, responsibility for the whole sorry financial mess can be pinned upon the pandemic, and the finger of blame pointed at the lockdowns it necessitated.

The economic results of the lockdowns are going to be catastrophic, but the seeds for financial catastrophe were sown long before this current crisis developed.

If magical misdirection is what is currently playing out, then once again there is the possibility that the timing of events is merely coincidental. However, a darker possibility is that desperate times call for desperate measures, and an engineered crisis was deemed necessary before financial disaster struck, so that fingers could be pointed at a suitable scapegoat.

Power, money and control

It's possible to go much deeper into the dark rabbit warren of conjecture.

I'll group all other potential motivations here, as it really is impossible to sort truth from lies, fact from fiction, and conspiracy theories from realistic possibilities.

Once again, I'd like to point out that I am not putting any of these ideas forward as my suggestion for what is going on, nor do I have any idea on how to assess the weight of probability of any particular scenario being likely to be correct.

I merely offer the wide range of ideas considered by some to be our current reality.

Just a few suggestions from a wealth of theories available online:

- Shifting more power and money to the 1%.
- A cashless society, world taxation, and loss of freedom.
- Dealing with environmental issues by restricting travel.
- Population control in a world with too many people.
- A prison planet ruled by a tiny elite.

I'll leave you to do your own research and reach your own conclusions.

The websites listed in **Appendix A: Resources** should give you a few good starting points.

The Great Reset

I don't intend to go too deep here, but just want to point you in the direction of the World Economic Forum (WEF)[84], and their openly stated desire for a "Great Reset".[85]

The WEF is like a Who's Who of world elite players who meet in Davos, Switzerland, flying in on their private jets for annual meetings to plan for our future. Fronted by Klaus Schwab, their mission statement begins as follows[86]:

> The Forum engages the foremost political, business, cultural and other leaders of society to shape global, regional and industry agendas.

These "foremost leaders" at the WEF who "shape global agendas" see the pandemic as an opportunity to accelerate their Great Reset goals[87]:

> As we enter a unique window of opportunity to shape the recovery, this initiative will offer insights to help inform all those determining the future state of global relations, the direction of national economies, the priorities of societies, the nature of business models and the management of a global commons. Drawing from the vision and vast expertise of the leaders engaged across the Forum's communities, the Great Reset initiative has a set of dimensions to build a new social contract that honours the dignity of every human being.

A recent video they produced highlighted their "8 predictions for 2030". The first line suggested "You'll own nothing... and you'll be happy."

This was followed by the idea that, "Whatever you want you'll rent... and it will be delivered by drone".

So wait a minute, if I own nothing and will rent it, who will own everything, so that I can rent it from them? I'm guessing that will be you and your billionaire buddies, Klaus?

---

[84] https://www.weforum.org/

[85] https://www.weforum.org/great-reset

[86] https://www.weforum.org/about/world-economic-forum

[87] https://www.weforum.org/great-reset

The video attracted a lot of negative attention, and surprise surprise, has now been removed from the WEF website. Fortunately it is still available on YouTube here:
https://www.youtube.com/watch?v=svyCzsenOnU

This article from the off-guardian.org website[88] provides an interesting overview of the Great Reset:

ARTICLE: "Own Nothing and Be Happy": The Great Reset's Vision of the Future

From the article's introduction:

> Driven by the vision of its influential CEO Klaus Schwab, the WEF is the main driving force for the dystopian 'great reset', a tectonic shift that intends to change how we live, work and interact with each other.
>
> The great reset entails a transformation of society resulting in permanent restrictions on fundamental liberties and mass surveillance as entire sectors are sacrificed to boost the monopoly and hegemony of pharmaceuticals corporations, high-tech/big data giants, Amazon, Google, major global chains, the digital payments sector, biotech concerns, etc.
>
> Using COVID-19 lockdowns and restrictions to push through this transformation, the great reset is being rolled out under the guise of a 'Fourth Industrial Revolution' in which older enterprises are to be driven to bankruptcy or absorbed into monopolies, effectively shutting down huge sections of the pre-COVID economy. Economies are being 'restructured' and many jobs will be carried out by AI-driven machines.

And its conclusion:

> The massive technocratic transformation currently envisaged regards humans as commodities to be controlled and monitored just like the lifeless technological drones and AI being promoted.
>
> But do not worry – you will be property-less and happy in your open prison of mass unemployment, state dependency, track and chip health passports, cashlessness, mass vaccination and dehumanisation.

---

[88] https://off-guardian.org/2020/11/12/own-nothing-and-be-happy-the-great-resets-vision-of-the-future/

The WEF was one of the three main co-hosts of "Event 201", the late 2019 pandemic simulation which was mentioned earlier in this book. The other co-hosts were The Bill & Melinda Gates Foundation, who are also one of WEF's major partners and Johns Hopkins Center for Health Security.

You can read more about these inter-connections here[89]:

ARTICLE: World Economic Forum: The Institution Behind 'The Great Reset'

> On examining the make up of Event 201, we find that the three institutions at the forefront of the simulation were the World Economic Forum, the Johns Hopkins Center for Health Security and the Bill and Melinda Gates Foundation.
>
> It is through the WEF that 'The Great Reset' was launched, in what the group said was in response to Covid-19. Johns Hopkins has been the go to source for the number of global infections and deaths thanks to their newly established 'Coronavirus Resource Center'. And then you have The Bill and Melinda Gates Foundation which has been a driving force behind efforts for a vaccination to be found and disseminated worldwide.

A quick look through the list of WEF Partners[90] finds all the global "usual suspects", including business leaders, politicians, royalty, big banks, pharma companies, food companies, oil companies, and many more influential figures.

Three companies that feature on the WEF Partners list:

- AstraZenica
- Moderna
- Pfizer

Oh dear. I'll let you do your own further research and draw your own conclusions, should this particular rabbit hole be of interest.

---

[89] https://stevenguinness2.wordpress.com/2020/07/08/world-economic-forum-a-look-at-the-institution-behind-the-great-reset/

[90] https://www.weforum.org/partners#search

Guessing games

So there are multiple possibilities on offer to explain what would appear to be an incredible over-reaction to something that seems to be only marginally worse than a particularly bad flu season. It really is impossible for us to know anything with any level of certainty, and as discussed, it would probably be wise to be very sceptical about anything anyone presents to you as being "the truth".

This leaves us in a tricky position, where it can feel like we are just playing guessing games, and wondering about possibilities.

A great piece of advice for judging a person's character and their motivations is to "Watch what they do, not what they say." This is also embodied in the familiar phrase, "Actions speak louder than words".

Perhaps it's better to actually listen to what they say, and then compare this to how they then behave. If these two observations are in conflict, then what they say is likely to be misleading, and their behaviour reveals true intent.

For example, politicians are at the head of the charge to get people inoculated. There are endless messages from our leaders promoting the positives. We have to protect our elderly and our frontline workers first. What about our leaders? Surely they should be at the front of the queue too, as we need them fit and healthy to be able to continue to perform the vital work they do?

How many politicians do we see or hear about getting vaccinated? How about the top executives in the big pharma companies? How keen are they to test out their own products?

Sometimes lack of action speaks louder than words too.

One final consideration, before we move on to look at vaccines in detail, is this. It doesn't seem unreasonable to assume that there are many more factors at play in this drama that we don't know about at all.

It is often said that there are four types of knowledge.

We know what we know: We know about the things we are familiar with, that are part of the world around us, that make up our own personal knowledge base. We are aware of this knowledge. Maybe you know about fixing plumbing problems, can speak Spanish, or have an in-depth knowledge of football scores.

We don't know what we know: There is another level of knowledge which is more subconscious. Our brains remember a lot more than we are aware of on a day-to-day basis. This is demonstrated when we take part in a quiz game, and can dredge all sorts of facts up in answer to obscure questions. Without being asked we are aware of this knowledge stored away in our mental filing cabinets.

We know what we don't know: We know other people can speak Chinese, mend cars and have an in-depth knowledge of ancient Roman history. We have an awareness of the gaps in our knowledge.

We don't know what we don't know: There is information and knowledge to which we have no access, and more importantly, have no awareness of its existence either.

This last area of information is the one most likely to blindside us, resulting in consequences that were completely unseen and unexpected. The phrase "we don't know what we don't know" is often attributed to Donald Rumsfelt, Secretary of Defense from 1975 to 1977 under Gerald Ford, and again from 2001 to 2006 under George W. Bush[91].

In response to questions on intelligence gathered about terrorist threats, he responded, "I feel that we know what we know and we don't know what we don't know."[92]

In terms of our current pandemic, we all believe there are things that we know. However, it is very reasonable to assume there are many things we don't know, and have no idea that this information even exists.

There will be a wide range of large companies, international agencies, government bodies and powerful individuals, perhaps some having competing interests, and others that may have goals in alignment with each other. We have no idea what goes on in the corridors of power or the boardrooms of mega-corporations. It is safe to assume that multiple decisions are made daily that will potentially impact on our individual lives and freedoms.

To question what is going on, to ponder possible ulterior motives behind the simple narrative we are fed would seem reasonable and rational. Surely this is what any sane, reasoning person does about most situations they come across in life?

We must not allow ourselves to be ridiculed or silenced into unquestioning acquiescence by those who would label anyone who would float a possibility that strays even slightly from the story we are being fed as "conspiracy theorists" or "anti-vaxxers"

---

[91] https://en.wikipedia.org/wiki/Donald_Rumsfeld

[92] https://www.urbandictionary.com/define.php ?term=We%20don%27t%20know%20what%20we%20don%27t%20know

PART 5: THE VACCINES WE TAKE

Reply when questioned on the safety of the polio vaccine he developed:
"It is safe, and you can't get safer than safe."

Jonas Salk

You can't get safer than safe

It would seem that vaccine makers have often been overly-confident in the safety of their products. Take, for example, the quote at the start of this section from Jonas Salk, creator of the polio vaccine... "You can't get safer than safe".

Unfortunately poor Jonas, I imagine, regretted his confident proclamation, as just a few short weeks later, as reported on history.com[93], disaster struck:

> Just weeks after the Salk vaccine had been declared safe, more than 200 polio cases were traced to lots contaminated with virulent live polio strains manufactured by the Cutter Laboratories in Berkeley, California. Most taken ill became severely paralyzed. Eleven died. In the haste to rush the vaccine to the public, the federal government had not provided proper supervision of the major drug companies contracted by the March of Dimes to produce 9 million doses of vaccine for 1955.

I'll just re-quote a short section from that article again, and see if you can see any modern-day parallels: "In the haste to rush the vaccine to the public, the federal government had not provided proper supervision of the major drug companies..."

And I'll refer again to the U.S. Department of Health and Human Services (HHS) Vaccine Adverse Event Reporting System (VAERS)[94], which to date (18th Feb 2021) lists 653 reports of "adverse reaction event" of "death" after taking a COVID-19 vaccine.

Only time will tell how safe our current COVID-19 vaccines will prove to be.

In the meantime, are you ready to be a guinea pig?

---

93 https://www.history.com/news/8-things-you-may-not-know-about-jonas-salk-and-the-polio-vaccine

94 https://vaers.hhs.gov/index.html

What is a vaccine?

From Wikipedia, a vaccine "is a biological preparation that provides active acquired immunity to a particular infectious disease. A vaccine typically contains a biological preparation from a disease-causing micro-organism, or since the beginning of the 21st century, made synthetically that resembles it. This preparation is often made from weakened or killed forms of the microbe, its toxins, or one of its surface proteins."[95]

The vaccine is designed to trigger the body's immune system to produce antibodies to the disease targeted, and thus prepare the body to react, should it meet the disease in the wild at some time in the future.

The aim of a vaccine is to ensure you have a better outcome if you are exposed to the virus. A vaccine doesn't stop you catching the disease. It pre-prepares your body so that it can mount an effective immune response to the virus.

Ultimately it is hoped that this will mean you have reduced symptoms, or no symptoms at all. It is also hoped that because you have a greatly reduced reaction to the virus you will not become infective, and will not pass on the virus to anybody else.

Thus, in theory, the virus is stopped in its tracks each time it infects a vaccinated person.

---

95 https://en.wikipedia.org/wiki/Vaccine

Vaccine history

In 1796 Edward Jenner took pus from the hand of a milkmaid with cowpox, scratched it into the arm of an 8-year-old boy, James Phipps, and six weeks later exposed James to smallpox, discovering that he didn't go on to develop the disease.

Jenner extended his studies and in 1798 reported that his vaccine was safe in children and adults.

In the 1880s Louis Pasteur developed vaccines for chicken cholera and anthrax.

In the early 1930s Alice Miles Woodruff and Ernest Goodpasture discovered that the fowlpox virus could be grown in embryonated chicken eggs. Other scientists followed, cultivating other viruses in eggs, leading to the development of a yellow fever vaccine in 1935 and a influenza vaccine in 1945.

There are three recognised generations of vaccines, as explained by Wikipedia[96]:

> First generation vaccines are whole-organism vaccines – either live and weakened, or killed forms. Live, attenuated vaccines, such as smallpox and polio vaccines, are able to induce killer T-cell (TC or CTL) responses, helper T-cell (TH) responses and antibody immunity. However, attenuated forms of a pathogen can convert to a dangerous form and may cause disease in immunocompromised vaccine recipients (such as those with AIDS). While killed vaccines do not have this risk, they cannot generate specific killer T cell responses and may not work at all for some diseases.
>
> Second generation vaccines were developed to reduce the risks from live vaccines. These are sub-unit vaccines, consisting of specific protein antigens (such as tetanus or diphtheria toxoid) or recombinant protein components (such as the hepatitis B surface antigen). They can generate TH and antibody responses, but not killer T cell responses.
>
> RNA vaccines and DNA vaccines are examples of third generation vaccines. In 2016 a DNA vaccine for the Zika virus began testing at the National Institutes of Health. Separately, Inovio Pharmaceuticals and GeneOne Life Science began tests of a

---

[96] https://en.wikipedia.org/wiki/Vaccine#History

> different DNA vaccine against Zika in Miami. Manufacturing the vaccines in volume was unsolved as of 2016. Clinical trials for DNA vaccines to prevent HIV are underway. mRNA vaccines such as BNT162b2 were developed in the year 2020 with the help of Operation Warp Speed and massively deployed to combat the coronavirus pandemic.

The current vaccines available for the SARS-CoV-2 coronavirus are both second generation (AstraZenica) and third generation (Pfizer and Moderna).

Let's take a look at each of these vaccines in a little more detail.

The current vaccines on offer

In the West, at time of writing (February 2021), there are three vaccines being widely used. The first to be announced comes from the Pfizer/BioNTech partnership, who stated on 9th November 2020, in their first interim analysis from their Phase 3 study[97]:

> "Today is a great day for science and humanity. The first set of results from our Phase 3 COVID-19 vaccine trial provides the initial evidence of our vaccine's ability to prevent COVID-19," said Dr. Albert Bourla, Pfizer Chairman and CEO.

Within 2 days Pfizer announced it had reached an agreement to supply the EU with 200 million doses of its mRNA-based vaccine candidate, BNT162b2. It would seem that 9th November wasn't just "a great day for science and humanity", it was also a great day for Pfizer and BioNTech share prices, which jumped by 12.5% and 18.2% respectively as markets opened[98].

The second announcement, this time from Moderna, came hot on the heels of the Pfizer press release. On the same day Pfizer released details of its EU deal, 11th November, Moderna published the first of several releases[99], with the news being announced that they had reached the primary endpoint of Phase 3 studies on 16th November.

Their enthusiastic statement[100] reads as follows:

> "This is a pivotal moment in the development of our COVID-19 vaccine candidate. Since early January, we have chased this virus with the intent to protect as many people around the world as possible. All along, we have known that each day matters. This positive interim analysis from our Phase 3 study has given us the first clinical validation that our vaccine can prevent COVID-19 disease, including severe disease," said Stéphane Bancel, Chief Executive Officer of Moderna.

---

[97] https://www.pfizer.com/news/press-release/press-release-detail/pfizer-and-biontech-announce-vaccine-candidate-against

[98] https://www.fool.com/investing/2020/11/09/why-pfizer-and-biontech-stocks-are-soaring-today/

[99] https://investors.modernatx.com/news-releases

[100] https://investors.modernatx.com/news-releases/news-release-details/modernas-covid-19-vaccine-candidate-meets-its-primary-efficacy

So wait a minute... Moderna had been "chasing the virus" since early January? The WHO tweet of 14th January declared "no clear evidence of human-to-human transmission". The WHO didn't categorize the crisis a a "Public Health Emergency of International Concern" (PHEIC) at their 23rd January meeting, waiting until the end of the month to do so. It wasn't until 11th March the outbreak was classified as a pandemic. Good to know that Moderna, a company which to that point had never produced a vaccine or medicine approved for use[101], were on the case so early!

A few days later, on 17th November, a follow-up press release from Moderna[102] informed us that the UK Government didn't plan to hang around, and needed no further evidence of efficacy.

A supply agreement had been made between two parties, and the press release suggested that this could result in the Moderna vaccine mRNA-1273 being "available to the UK population as early as March 2021", if approved for use, of course, by UK regulatory authorities.

On Tuesday 8th December, less than a month after the UK/Moderna supply agreement had been made, Margaret Keenan, a 90-year-old grandmother from Northern Ireland, became the first person in the world to receive the Pfizer COVID-19 vaccine, outside of a trial[103].

It would seem that the vaccine manufacturers had no problems with the UK regulatory authorities, and Moderna's own estimate of "as early as March 2021" was woefully pessimistic. By early December, less than one month after the initial announcements of completion of Phase 3 trial analysis, needles were going into arms. By the end of January 2021, millions of people around the world had already received their first jab.

As if the news wasn't already good enough in early November, another player joined the party. The AstraZenica partnership with Oxford University had been announced on the AstraZenica website on 30th April 2020[104], so they did very well to make their "effective vaccine" claim just 2 weeks after Pfizer and Moderna made their announcements.

---

101 https://www.modernatx.com/pipeline

102 https://investors.modernatx.com/news-releases/news-release-details/moderna-announces-supply-agreement-united-kingdom-government

103 https://www.reuters.com/article/uk-health-coronavirus-britain-idUSKBN28I0OQ

104 https://www.astrazeneca.com/media-centre/press-releases/2020/astrazeneca-and-oxford-university-announce-landmark-agreement-for-covid-19-vaccine.html

On 23rd November AstraZenica announced[105]: "Positive high-level results from an interim analysis of clinical trials of AZD1222 in the UK and Brazil showed the vaccine was highly effective in preventing COVID-19, the primary endpoint, and no hospitalisations or severe cases of the disease were reported in participants receiving the vaccine."

From the date of their partnership announcement on the last day of April to the positive news at the end of November, it took the Oxford Uni/AstraZenica team less than 7 months to produce a vaccine that was, as far as the UK Government was concerned, ready for roll-out.

The initial "best-case-scenario" timeline of "12 to 18 months" turned out to be wildly inaccurate. 7 months was all it took to achieve something that had never before been done in the history of medicine.

---

105 https://www.astrazeneca.com/content/astraz/media-centre/press-releases/2020/azd1222hlr.html

Virus vectors vs. mRNA

The AstraZenica vaccine uses tried-and-tested vaccine technology. Known as a virus vector, these types of vaccines have been used for decades. The vaccine uses a virus, usually modified to be relatively harmless, to encourage the body to mount a defensive response. This prepares the body in advance, so that if it then encounters the real virus it is ready with the immune response blueprint to fight back effectively.

In simple terms, the vaccine is designed to mimic the virus it is hoping to protect against, and train the body's immune system to react accordingly if a person is later infected by the actual virus.

To create flu and coronavirus vaccines an adenovirus is usually used. This is a common virus that can, according to the CDC website[106], "cause cold-like symptoms, fever, sore throat, bronchitis, pneumonia, diarrhea, and pink eye (conjunctivitis)". The common cold, for example, is caused by an adenovirus. The adenovirus is used to prompt the body to mount its defence.

The AstraZenica vaccine is based on a modified chimpanzee adenovirus.

Pfizer and Moderna use a different type of vaccine technology called Messenger RNA, or mRNA. This new technique uses genetic material made in the lab, which is designed to cause your body to make a certain part of a virus. In the case of the COVID-19 vaccines, they cause the body to create the SARS-CoV-2 virus spike proteins. Then, similar to the virus vector vaccines, your body mounts an immune response to these intruders, and is thus prepared when (or if) the actual virus is encountered.

There are a couple of points worth noting here about mRNA vaccines.

1) They have NEVER been approved for use in humans before now, so with the hurried approval for emergency use, and the hasty vaccine roll-out, they are still classified as experimental, even on the manufacturers' websites[107]:
   From the Moderna website: "The Moderna COVID-19 Vaccine has not been approved or licensed by the US Food and Drug Administration (FDA), but has been authorized for emergency use by FDA, under an Emergency Use Authorization (EUA), to prevent Coronavirus Disease 2019 (COVID-19) for use in

---

106 https://www.cdc.gov/adenovirus/index.html

107 https://www.modernatx.com/covid19vaccine-eua/providers/

individuals 18 years of age and older. There is no FDA-approved vaccine to prevent COVID-19."

2) Much is still unknown about how they will work.
    a. How long will immunity last?
    b. Will they halt onward transmission of the disease?
    c. Will further "booster doses" be necessary?
    d. Will they be effective against virus variants?
3) Moderna, leading the mRNA vaccine charge, has never produced a previously approved vaccine or medication... ever.
4) AstraZenica, on the other hand, have had many traditional vaccines approved, but have no mRNA products.108 However, between 2013 and 2016 they invested $380million in Moderna, resulting in ownership of a 9% stake of the company. That stake is currently worth around $2billion.109

By taking any of these experimental vaccines we are de-facto enrolled as part of a worldwide study group. Let's hope it goes well.

If you want a (relatively) easy-to-understand explanation of these vaccine technologies, and others, this article is very informative:
https://theconversation.com/from-adenoviruses-to-rna-the-pros-and-cons-of-different-covid-vaccine-technologies-145454

Published on 18th September 2020, it is interesting to note that the article raises the suggestion that one of the challenges faced by mRNA vaccines is "they are likely to face considerable regulatory hurdles before being approved for use".

It seems these hurdles were easily surmounted.

Two other potential hurdles for mRNA vaccines mentioned in the same article are:

- As they only allow a fragment of the virus to be made, they may prompt a poor protective immune response, meaning multiple boosters may be needed.
- There is a theoretical probability vaccine DNA can integrate into your genome.

---

[108] https://www.astrazeneca.com/our-therapy-areas/pipeline.html

[109] https://www.thetimes.co.uk/article/astrazeneca-investment-in-moderna-hits-2bn-as-vaccine-hopes-soar-pjt3x3lpl

It seems there is a lot we don't know, particularly about this "next generation" of mRNA vaccines.

Are you happy to be a participant in on-going trials for new experimental vaccine technology?

Emergency Use Authorizations (EUA)

So how did the vaccine roll-out progress with such speed? In the UK it seemed that the government was ready to accept without question the first vaccines announced, and were keen to begin the immunisation program as soon as possible. Margaret Keenan received her first jab while most other European countries wanted to wait for more safety data.

In the USA, Emergency Use Authorization (EUA) was granted for the Pfizer vaccine on 11th December. Margaret Keenan had already been back at home in Northern Ireland for a couple of days after her jab by this point, making the U.S. look overly-zealously cautious in the global rush to round up the population and begin "getting back to normal".

From the FDA (U.S. Food & Drug Administration) website[110], here is what "emergency use authorization" means:

> Under section 564 of the Federal Food, Drug, and Cosmetic Act (FD&C Act), the FDA Commissioner may allow **unapproved medical products** or unapproved uses of approved medical products to be used in an emergency **to diagnose, treat, or prevent serious or life-threatening diseases** or conditions caused by CBRN threat agents **when there are no adequate, approved, and available alternatives**. [emphasis added]

As an interesting aside, I had to do a quick search elsewhere to find out what CBRN threat agents are. Down the acronym rabbit-hole... From the CPNI (Centre for the Protection of the National Infrastructure) website[111]:

"'CBRN' is the abbreviation commonly used to describe the malicious use of Chemical, Biological, Radiological and Nuclear materials or weapons with the intention to cause significant harm or disruption."

So, the key takeaway here is that the vaccines are "unapproved", but are allowed to be used under an EUA to prevent serious or life-threatening diseases, when there are no alternatives.

The FDA granted an EUA for the Moderna mRNA vaccine on 18th December 2020[112], a week after Pfizer's EUA.

---

110 https://www.fda.gov/emergency-preparedness-and-response/mcm-legal-regulatory-and-policy-framework/emergency-use-authorization

111 https://www.cpni.gov.uk/chemical-biological-radiological-and-nuclear-cbrn-threats-0

To date, AstraZenica hasn't received EUA in The States. According to TheHill website[113], this isn't likely to happen until April 2021.

ARTICLE: AstraZeneca vaccine likely won't be authorized in U.S. until April

> "We project, if everything goes well, that the readout and emergency use authorization may be granted somewhere early in the month of April," Moncef Slaoui, the chief science adviser for the administration's Operation Warp Speed, told reporters.

BusinessInsider website[114] suggests this is, in part, because some aspects of the AstraZeneca trial didn't quite go to plan.

ARTICLE: When will AstraZeneca's COVID-19 vaccine be available in the US?

> The AstraZeneca trial also included at least one big mistake. A subset of trial participants under 55 years old were accidentally administered a half-dose first shot, followed by a full-strength second jab.
>
> "That's a pretty serious error," Dr. Cody Meissner, chief of pediatric infectious disease at Tufts Medical Center, and one of the vaccine experts on the FDA's advisory committee, told Insider of the mishap.

In fine UK Daily Mail style[115], outrage at the FDA snub for our fine British vaccine was expressed in no uncertain terms. They were keen to point out that the AstraZenica vaccine was "cheaper and easier to store than other COVID-19 shots such as those manufactured by Pfizer and Moderna".

---

[112] https://www.fda.gov/emergency-preparedness-and-response/coronavirus-disease-2019-covid-19/moderna-covid-19-vaccine

[113] https://thehill.com/policy/healthcare/532163-astrazeneca-vaccine-likely-wont-be-authorized-in-us-until-april

[114] https://www.businessinsider.com/when-will-astrazeneca-covid-vaccine-be-approved-in-us-2021-1

[115] https://www.dailymail.co.uk/health/article-9102431/Doctor-slams-FDA-not-approving-AstraZenecas-coronavirus-vaccine.html

ARTICLE: Johns Hopkins professor claims the real reason why U.S. won't approve simpler Oxford-AstraZeneca vaccine is because the 'turtle' FDA is a 'broke federal bureaucracy' of 17,000 people that are just 'too slow'

> A doctor has slammed the U.S. Food and Drug Administration (FDA) for not approving AstraZeneca-University of Oxford's coronavirus vaccine.
>
> On Wednesday, Great Britain became the fist [sic] country in the world to grant authorization to the COVID-19 jab.
>
> The vaccine holds great appeal because it's inexpensive - costing $3 to $4 per dose - and can be stored in refrigerators for up to six months rather than at ultra-cold temperatures required for other vaccines.
>
> However, a top Trump administration official has said Americans will likely not receive AstraZeneca's coronavirus shot before April - three months after the U.K.'s green light.
>
> Dr Marty Makary, a professor in the School of Medicine at Johns Hopkins University Bloomberg School of Public Health, took to Twitter to blast the decision and said the FDA's slow-moving 'bureaucracy' - not worries over safety - are the real reason for the delay.

Perhaps "cheaper and easier" is why the UK Government hastily approved the AstraZenica jab for emergency use in the UK on 30th December, despite the in-trial mistakes.

The big rush

In the early stages of the pandemic, the oft-touted timeline for vaccine creation was "12 to 18 months" as a minimum, perhaps longer. The first vaccine announcement came well within the most optimistic estimate, and more announcements followed in quick succession.

Moderna's announcement, coupled with its agreement with the UK government, suggested vaccines could be administered "as early as March 2021". The first shot (Pfizer) was given on 8th December 2020, less than a month after the first vaccine announcement, at least 3 months ahead of the pharma giant's optimistic best guess.

By the end of January, less than two short months later, millions of jabs have been given, despite the fact that no real mid-term or long-term safety data is available, and despite the fact that there are still many unanswered questions around the safety and efficacy of these hastily produced vaccines, and despite the fact they are still only classified as unapproved and experimental.

Especially concerning are the unanswered questions around the "next generation" of mRNA vaccines, yet these seem to be the ones to receive the quickest approvals, and the fastest roll-outs.

How have these vaccines achieved such widespread acceptance so quickly? Do we have ourselves to blame, at least to some degree?

Dr. Vernon Coleman suggests this is one factor at play in his book "Vaccines Are Dangerous – And Don't Work"[116]:

> The idea of vaccination... is very easy to sell to people. And it is enormously profitable for drug companies and doctors.
>
> People love vaccination because it promises them an easy way to avoid illness without having to do anything themselves. They want to believe that it works and they want to believe that it is safe. It is for this reason that vaccines against just about everything (including obesity) are being introduced.

---

116 https://www.amazon.com/Vaccines-Are-Dangerous-Dont-Work-ebook/dp/B00HSSRK1E/

A small matter of liability

In 1986 in The States the National Childhood Vaccine Injury Act was introduced.

From Wikipedia[117]:

> The National Childhood Vaccine Injury Act (NCVIA) of 1986 was signed into law by United States President Ronald Reagan as part of a larger health bill on November 14, 1986. NCVIA's purpose was to eliminate the potential financial liability of vaccine manufacturers due to vaccine injury claims to ensure a stable market supply of vaccines, and to provide cost-effective arbitration for vaccine injury claims. Under the NCVIA, the National Vaccine Injury Compensation Program (NVICP) was created to provide a federal no-fault system for compensating vaccine-related injuries or death by establishing a claim procedure involving the United States Court of Federal Claims and special masters.

This meant that vaccine manufacturers could no longer be taken to court over claims that their products had resulted in injury, harm or death. Instead the Federal Government was now on the hook to pay out any damages awarded in court.

The Wikipedia article is surprisingly short, for such an important, and currently very relevant topic. Let's look elsewhere for further information.

A good starting point would be to find and watch a drama/documentary from last year called "1986: The Act (2020)"[118], a dramatic forensic examination of the 1986 National Childhood Vaccine Injury Act and its consequences.

Here's a good in-depth article from The Atlantic[119], published in 2019:

ARTICLE: Why the Government Pays Billions to People Who Claim Injury by Vaccines

The article begins:

---

117 https://en.wikipedia.org/wiki/National_Childhood_Vaccine_Injury_Act

118 https://www.imdb.com/title/tt12708236/

119 https://www.theatlantic.com/health/archive/2019/05/vaccine-safety-program/589354/

> "Vaccines are safe," says Narayan Nair. "That's the message we need to get out there."
>
> Nair is a physician. He is also the head of the Vaccine Injury Compensation Program—the system through which the U.S. government has, over the past three decades, paid more than $4 billion to people who claim to have been harmed by vaccines.
>
> According to its public record, from 2013 to 2017 alone, the program paid out an average of $229 million a year to patients and their families. The average payment was about $430,000.

Let's just pause here... Vaccines are causing harm, people are claiming in court, but not against the pharma companies who made the vaccines, as the manufacturers are protected by the 1986 NCVIA (National Childhood Vaccine Injury Act) ruling. The government is paying out millions of dollars in compensation via the NVICP (National Vaccine Injury Compensation Program). No, wait, let's correct that... the government is compensating victims with taxpayer money. The pharma companies are fully indemnified against any liability.

The article continues:

> The fact that the government pays hundreds of millions of dollars every year to people who claim they've been injured by vaccines could be an alarming thing to see in your Facebook News Feed, especially if you're a parent whose pediatrician assured you that vaccination is nothing to worry about. In one case, a viral article called "Flu Vaccine Is the Most Dangerous Vaccine in the U.S. Based on Settled Cases for Injuries" points to these payments as evidence of vaccines' danger.

Here's a September 2010 article from CBSnews.com[120] which details a payout for autism suspected to have resulted from vaccination, despite reams of "evidence" suggesting there is no such link.

ARTICLE: Family to Receive $1.5M+ in First-Ever Vaccine-Autism Court Award

> The first court award in a vaccine-autism claim is a big one. CBS News has learned the family of Hannah Poling will receive more than $1.5 million dollars for her life care; lost earnings; and pain and suffering for the first year alone.

---

[120] https://www.cbsnews.com/news/family-to-receive-15m-plus-in-first-ever-vaccine-autism-court-award/

> In addition to the first year, the family will receive more than \$500,000 per year to pay for Hannah's care. Those familiar with the case believe the compensation could easily amount to \$20 million over the child's lifetime.

About 4,800 similar cases await trial:

> In acknowledging Hannah's injuries, the government said vaccines aggravated an unknown mitochondrial disorder Hannah had which didn't "cause" her autism, but "resulted" in it. It's unknown how many other children have similar undiagnosed mitochondrial disorder. All other autism "test cases" have been defeated at trial. Approximately 4,800 are awaiting disposition in federal vaccine court.

The CDC still denies any link:

> Then-director of the Centers for Disease Control Julie Gerberding (who is now President of Merck Vaccines) stated: "The government has made absolutely no statement indicating that vaccines are a cause of autism. This does not represent anything other than a very specific situation and a very sad situation as far as the family of the affected child."

Two quick points to note here:

1. The government says the vaccine didn't cause autism, but resulted in it. That sounds like a very fine-line distinction to make to avoid admitting an actual causal link. Blaming an "unknown mitochondrial disorder" suggests they just don't know, but need a scapegoat.
2. The CDC director went on to become president of Merck Vaccines. It is commonly suggested that influence over the government by big pharma lobbying, facilitated by those in top level positions within government departments, is later rewarded with a high salary position within the pharma industry after retirement from government "service".

I'd urge you to read the full article here:
https://www.cbsnews.com/news/family-to-receive-15m-plus-in-first-ever-vaccine-autism-court-award/

So why is the 1986 Act relevant today?

Well, the situation is exactly the same now in the USA with the COVID vaccines. This CNBC article[121] explains:

ARTICLE: You can't sue Pfizer or Moderna if you have severe Covid vaccine side effects. The government likely won't compensate you for damages either

> KEY POINTS
>
> - Under the PREP Act, companies like Pfizer and Moderna have total immunity from liability if something unintentionally goes wrong with their vaccines.
> - A little-known government program provides benefits to people who can prove they suffered serious injury from a vaccine.
> - That program rarely pays, covering just 29 claims over the last decade.

The article continues:

> If you experience severe side effects after getting a Covid vaccine, lawyers tell CNBC there is basically no one to blame in a U.S. court of law.
>
> The federal government has granted companies like Pfizer and Moderna immunity from liability if something unintentionally goes wrong with their vaccines.
>
> You also can't sue the Food and Drug Administration for authorizing a vaccine for emergency use, nor can you hold your employer accountable if they mandate inoculation as a condition of employment.

Here is what the PREP (Public Readiness and Emergency Preparedness) Act means:

> In February, Health and Human Services Secretary Alex Azar invoked the Public Readiness and Emergency Preparedness Act. The 2005 law empowers the HHS secretary to provide legal protection to companies making or distributing critical medical supplies, such as vaccines and treatments, unless there's "willful misconduct" by the company. The protection lasts until 2024.

---

[121] https://www.cnbc.com/amp/2020/12/16/covid-vaccine-side-effects-compensation-lawsuit.html

> That means that for the next four years, these companies "cannot be sued for money damages in court" over injuries related to the administration or use of products to treat or protect against Covid.

Why would the government do that?:

> Dunn thinks a big reason for the unprecedented protection has to do with the expedited timeline.
>
> "When the government said, 'We want you to develop this four or five times faster than you normally do,' most likely the manufacturers said to the government, 'We want you, the government, to protect us from multimillion-dollar lawsuits,'" said Dunn.

All of this begs the most obvious question:

If the vaccines are as safe and effective as the manufacturers claim, why would they feel they need immunity from any financial liability?

Surely this sort of blanket protection takes away the incentive to be absolutely rigorous about vaccine safety.

The situation is very similar in the UK. From legal website jurist.org[122]:

ARTICLE: UK government grants Pfizer civil legal indemnity for COVID-19 vaccine

> The UK government announced Thursday that it had granted Pfizer legal indemnity protecting the American pharmaceutical company from civil lawsuits due to any unforeseen complications arising from problems with its COVID-19 vaccine. The special legal indemnity was the result of an emergency government consultation in September, when the UK Department of Health & Social Care determined that changes to civil liability were necessary to better facilitate the widespread use of a COVID-19 vaccine in Britain.

Personally I don't see how granting the manufacturer full legal indemnity "better facilitates the widespread use of a vaccine". Do you?

If the vaccines are as safe as the manufacturers claim, let them take full responsibility if anything does go wrong.

---

[122] https://www.jurist.org/news/2020/12/uk-government-grants-pfizer-civil-legal-indemnity-for-covid-19-vaccine/

Fingers crossed...

Here is a list of some assumptions you are making, or hopes you have, when you reach decision point of accepting a COVID-19 experimental vaccine shot:

1) Vaccines in general are safe and desirable.
2) The coronavirus vaccine you are about to have has been tested thoroughly, is safe, and contains nothing potentially harmful to you.
3) The vaccine you receive will be effective at preventing you becoming ill if you do get infected by the virus at some point in the future.
4) The vaccine will stop transmission of the virus, or at least reduce it, from you to other people.
5) The pharma companies producing the vaccines can be trusted, and have your health as their main priority.
6) The government encouraging you to come in for your shot also has your best interests at heart.
7) The medical pros encouraging you to get inoculated have all the info they need to make informed decisions and provide reliable advice.

And here are a few other points to think about:

- The vaccines have already shown some side effects in some recipients, sometimes within minutes. Is this a risk you are prepared to take?
- All vaccine trials, due to the nature of the hurried roll-out, have produced only short-term safety and efficacy results. How about mid-term safety?
- Are there any long-term safety issues that we don't yet know about? Don't forget, the big pharma companies take no responsibility if anything goes wrong.
- Are you going to need to be vaccinated every year, if the virus mutates, or if immunity reduces over time?
- Will having the vaccine change how you can behave on a day-to-day basis? Will it allow us to eventually "get back to normal"?
- Will you need a vaccine to travel in the future? There is already lots of chatter in the media about "vaccine certificates" or "vaccine passports".

Questions to ask

Are you still on the fence? That's OK if you are. There is a lot to consider here.

If you're still wavering, then I'd like to point you to this wonderful little article by Kit Knightly[123]:

ARTICLE: 5 questions to ask your friends who plan to get the Covid vaccine

Kit begins by pointing out:

> Many of us have friends or family who plan on getting the vaccine. Maybe they truly believe they are in danger. Maybe they think it's better safe than sorry. Maybe they just want to be able to go to the pub again.
>
> If you know someone who is planning on getting vaccinated against Covid19, ask them these five questions. Make sure they understand exactly what they're asking for.

The questions to ask are as follows, with fully detailed answers available by reading the article:
https://off-guardian.org/2021/02/15/5-questions-to-ask-your-friends-who-plan-to-get-the-covid-vaccine/

1. Did you know that we have never successfully vaccinated against any coronavirus?
2. Did you know it usually takes 5 to 10 years to fully develop a vaccine?
3. Did you know that the COVID "vaccine" is based on new technology, which has never been approved for use on humans before?
4. Did you know that the pharmaceutical companies can't be sued if the vaccine hurts or kills someone?
5. Did you know 99.8% of people survive COVID-19?

---

[123] https://off-guardian.org/2021/02/15/5-questions-to-ask-your-friends-who-plan-to-get-the-covid-vaccine/

If you've already made your decision to avoid being vaccinated, then this set of questions might be useful when you meet the inevitable challenges you'll face from those who think you are "being irresponsible" and "endangering others".

Or, may I humbly suggest, you could give a copy of this book to your argumentative challengers and propose that they ask themselves some questions and do some critical thinking of their own before jumping to a hasty decision and condemning you for not following the herd.

PART 6: THE WINNERS WE CREATE

"Winners have no interest or association in the opinions, actions or affairs of losers."

Jeffrey Fry

Means, motive and opportunity

In any crime novel or TV cop show drama the detective trying to track down the killer must look for someone who has the timeless triumvirate of criminal intent: means, motive and opportunity.

First of all, the potential criminal must have the actual ability to have committed the murder. Next, without a reason for the crime, it is hard to understand why the accused is the likely perpetrator. Finally, the suspect must have also had the opportunity to commit the deadly deed.

If any one of these factors is missing from the prosecutor's case, a conviction, under an assumption of "innocent until proven guilty" guidelines, is much less likely.

So what is the "crime" that has been, or is being committed here?

Once again, I have to point out that all of this is based on looking at the actions certain groups of people take, and wondering about potential outcomes from those actions. This leads us to considering motives behind the actions.

So we're not looking at your standard "body-on-the-floor-outlined-by-chalk" murder case. This is more of a "missing-presumed-dead" situation, where a suspected crime has been committed, but as yet we have neither the dead body nor the smoking gun.

Like any case of this nature, it is possible that the "victim" re-appears none the worse for wear after going on a bit of a bender, but it is also possible that there is a body in a shallow grave in the woods just waiting to be discovered.

Our simplest "undiscovered-body-in-a-shallow-grave-in-the-woods" scenario isn't to difficult to imagine. We've already looked at giant pharma companies, and considered the money and influence they have over government policy. Their past track record of profiteering and buying influence makes them an obvious first suspect.

The two vaccines that have been approved for use in the USA under Emergency Use Authorizations are only supposed to be cleared for such use if there is no alternative treatment. Both hydroxychloroquine (HCQ) and ivermectin have, according to many doctors, been proven to be very effective, both in prophylactic use, and as early treatment of COVID-19. There are many trials which would appear to demonstrate this effectiveness.

Yet any quick search on Google would seem to suggest the opposite, as do guidelines of many medical advisors to governments around the world.

Hydroxychloroquine

Dr. Simone Gold's book, "I Do Not Consent"[124], argues the case for hydroxychloroquine very strongly. She also explains how HCQ, according to many media sources, changed from being considered a very safe drug that has been used for decades and had billions of doses given, to a dangerous drug with serious potential to cause heart arrhythmia.

She is backed by dozens of doctors who have come together to form America's Frontline Doctors group:
https://www.americasfrontlinedocs.com/

Dr. Gold suggests in her book that a complete course of HCQ therapy for treatment of COVID-19 would cost less than USD $10.

Here's another report from a doctor, Dr.Joseph Mercola[125] on how effective HCQ is at dealing with the disease if used as an early treatment, ideally within the first 5 days of onset of symptoms:

ARTICLE: NY Doctor Proved Everyone Wrong About Hydroxychloroquine

Story at a glance:

- As early as March 2020, Dr. Vladimir Zelenko boasted a near-100% success rate treating COVID-19 patients with hydroxychloroquine (HCQ), azithromycin and zinc sulfate for five days
- Zelenko has now treated 3,000 patients with COVID-19 symptoms and only three high-risk patients have died
- Misinformation and outright lies were spun about HCQ, including fabricated research, in an apparent effort to suppress and prevent widespread use
- Early treatment is crucial. During the first five days of SARS-CoV-2 infection, the viral load remains fairly steady. Around Day 5, it exponentially increases, potentially overwhelming your immune system. To prevent complications, treatment needs to begin within the first five days of symptom onset

---

[124] https://www.amazon.com/Do-Not-Consent-Against-Medical-ebook/dp/B08L8JK7FL/

[125] https://articles.mercola.com/sites/articles/archive/2021/02/07/hydroxychloroquine-for-covid.aspx

- Early treatment is also crucial to prevent "long-haul" symptoms after recovery. None of Zelenko's patients who started their treatment within the first five days went on to develop long-haul symptoms

And this website[126] pulls together data from, to date, 249 studies on HCQ effectiveness, of which 179 are peer reviewed, and of which 205 compare treatment and control groups. The evidence they present is pretty conclusive. HCQ appears to be very effective if prescribed early enough.

Ivermectin

Ivermectin has similarly strong credentials, and there are many studies supporting claims that ivermectin is even more effective than HCQ, both for prophylactic use, for early stage COVID-19 cases, and even for later stage infections.

Dr. Pierre Kory testified on 8th December 2020 at the U.S. Senate Committee on Homeland Security and Governmental Affairs, and you can see his impassioned presentation, posted on YouTube by Senator Ron Johnson.
https://www.youtube.com/watch?v=YgOAaLmoa68

You can see the entire hearing, entitled "Early Out Patient Treatment: An Essential Part of a COVID-19 Solution, Part II" at the U.S. Senate Committee Homeland Security and Governmental Affairs website here:
https://www.hsgac.senate.gov/early-outpatient-treatment-an-essential-part-of-a-covid-19-solution-part-ii

If you don't have time to spare the 2 hours 50 minutes to watch the entire hearing, I strongly urge you to invest 8 minutes of your life to watch the YouTube clip of Dr. Kory's talk. If you want to see Dr. Kory's presentation within the full senate hearing video, Senator Johnson introduces him at the 49:00 minute mark.

Dr. Kory is also backed by a large group of peers who share the same message. You can find out more at the Front Line COVID-19 Critical Care Alliance (FLCCC) website, here:
https://covid19criticalcare.com/

Ivermectin, like hydroxychloroquine, is an off-patent drug, meaning any licensed pharma company can produce it, which makes it very cheap. The profits on these drugs are marginal at best, when compared to newly patented drugs, such as the much touted, but somewhat ineffective

---

126 https://c19study.com/

remdesivir. Or when compared to the profit margins on newly patented vaccines!

From the FLCCC website[127]:

> In March, 2020 we first published our MATH+ Treatment Protocol for COVID-19, intended for hospitalized patients. The recently developed I-MASK+ Prophylaxis & Early Outpatient Treatment Protocol for COVID-19 is instead directed for use as a prophylaxis and in early outpatient treatment after contracting COVID-19. The protocols thus complement each other, and both are physiologic-based combination treatment regimens developed by leaders in critical care medicine. **All component medicines are FDA-approved, inexpensive, readily available and have been used for decades with well-established safety profiles.** [emphasis added]

Once again, there is a great resource that draws together data from many trials using ivermectin to treat COVID-19. To date they have details of 59 studies, 22 peer reviewed, 39 with results comparing treatment and control groups. Once again the evidence is strong that ivermectin is very effective in combating the effects of COVID-19.

Ivermectin Update: 14th January 2021

From the FLCCC website:

> Their [The U.S. National Institutes of Health (NIH)] recommendation has now been upgraded to the same level as those for widely used monoclonal antibodies & convalescent plasma, which is a "neither for nor against" recommendation. The significance of this change is that the NIH has decided to no longer recommend against the use of ivermectin in the treatment of COVID-19 by the nation's health care providers. A consequence of this change is that ivermectin has now been made a clear therapeutic option for patients.

So, to summarise, The U.S. National Institutes of Health (NIH), is no longer against the use of ivermectin, but equally is not for it either. But doctors are now free to prescribe if they choose to do so.

Did you see this news trumpeted in the press? I'm guessing not, as it was buried under the ever-ongoing avalanche of pro-vaccine rhetoric, and fear-mongering reports of case numbers, hospitalizations and deaths.

---

127 https://covid19criticalcare.com/

Did the NIH highlight the good news? Accessing the home page of the NIH website a couple of times over the last two weeks of January 2021 revealed nothing. The website has a scrolling swipe of five images linking to latest news and updates. On every visit to the site, at least two of these updates linked to positive COVID-19 vaccine news.

For example, on Sunday 31st January, the five main updates featured on the NIH home page, in order, were:

1) Janssen COVID-19 Vaccine Interim Results
   Single dose vaccine appears safe and effective at preventing moderate and severe COVID-19.
   https://www.nih.gov/news-events/news-releases/janssen-investigational-covid-19-vaccine-interim-analysis-phase-3-clinical-data-released
2) Vice President Harris at NIH
   Watch as Vice President Kamala Harris receives her second dose of the Moderna COVID-19 Vaccine at the NIH Clinical Center.
   https://videocast.nih.gov/watch=41481
3) NIH launches central COVID-19 website
   New resource for accurate information on vaccines, treatments and NIH-funded research.
   https://covid19.nih.gov/
4) Combat COVID
   Participate in a late phase clinical trial or donate plasma.
   https://combatcovid.hhs.gov/
5) January is Thyroid Awareness Month
   Hyperthyroidism, or overactive thyroid, affects around 1 out of 100 people in the U.S.
   https://www.niddk.nih.gov/health-information/endocrine-diseases/hyperthyroidism

That's a full 80% of the front page of the NIH headlines dedicated to positive or potentially positive news about COVID vaccines, or vaccine trials. The fact that it is Thyroid Awareness Month gets a brief look-in at the end.

Bear in mind that the NIH covers all medical issues. From their own "Who We Are" page, "The National Institutes of Health (NIH), a part of the U.S. Department of Health and Human Services, is the nation's medical research agency — making important discoveries that improve health and save lives."

There is not a single mention or link to the cheap, off-patent medicine, which has been used for decades, with a very good safety profile, having been authorised a potential option open to doctors to improve health and save lives.

A search of the NIH site for "ivermectin" produces this article as the first link:
https://www.covid19treatmentguidelines.nih.gov/antiviral-therapy/ivermectin/

On accessing this article on 31st January 2021 it can be seen it was last updated on 27th August 2020. At that time the article states, "We are currently updating the Ivermectin section of the Guidelines. Pending release of the updates, please see the COVID-19 Treatment Guidelines Panel's Statement on the Use of Ivermectin for the Treatment of COVID-19." Further down the article you can also discover that "The COVID-19 Treatment Guidelines Panel **recommends against** the use of **ivermectin** for the treatment of COVID-19, except in a clinical trial." [emphasis exactly as presented by NIH]

The Statement on the Use of Ivermectin link leads to the 14th January article which the FLCCC doctors reference in their update:
https://www.covid19treatmentguidelines.nih.gov/statement-on-ivermectin/

Here it clearly states, "The COVID-19 Treatment Guidelines Panel (the Panel) has determined that currently there are insufficient data to recommend either for or against the use of ivermectin for the treatment of COVID-19."

Strange, isn't it, that in more than 2 weeks since their own panel made new recommendations on potentially ground-breaking use of an incredibly cheap and safe drug the NIH hasn't managed to update its own main page on the use of ivermectin as a treatment for COVID-19.

If they are short on website maintenance staff, they could give me a login and password and I'll get it done in a couple of minutes for them.

Whodunnit?

In conclusion, it would appear that there are at least two potentially viable alternative treatments for COVID-19, yet there is a real lack of urgency from those in authority to approve these drugs as COVID-19 treatment options.

Tests and studies which appear to strongly support the claims by these groups of highly qualified doctors don't get anywhere near the same amount of media coverage as the ubiquitous publicity for vaccine development and roll-out.

One has to wonder, if there are real alternatives, not only for treatment, but potentially also in prevention, why these options are being ignored, even suppressed.

One possible conclusion that is easy to reach is that if these cheap, off-patent medicines were approved as COVID-19 treatments, under the FDA guidelines on EUA, there would be no grounds to continue to grant authorization for emergency use to the experimental vaccines currently being rolled-out with all possible haste.

So to return to our potential "undiscovered-body-in-a-shallow-grave-in-the-woods" scenario, it isn't hard to imagine that Big Pharma has the means (influence in government and the media), motive (billions of dollars) and the opportunity (a pandemic in urgent need of a solution), and thus becomes a credible suspect, when we consider why there is such a huge push towards vaccines, and away from any other alternative at all.

Follow the money

Another mantra often repeated on TV shows and in the movies, when the hero is trying to track down the most likely suspect, is the suggestion to "follow the money".

James Rickards has authored an enlightening series of books on the global economy, and the troubles he sees ahead.

He has spent time working on Wall Street, has acted as a top-level financial analyst for the CIA, helping construct and play out financial war game scenarios, and has spent time mixing with and interviewing global elite financiers in locations like Davos, high in the Swiss Alps. It is pretty safe to say that he knows more than most about international finances and world economy.

In his series of books he has pretty much been shouting from the rooftops that the global economy is currently very unstable. He suggests another crash, like those seen in 1997, 2000 and 2008, is inevitable. This time, he says, it will be bigger and much, much worse than anything that has happened before, as almost all asset classes have been blown into huge bubbles by central bank money printing policies.

He goes even further, suggesting that the world is long-overdue for another currency reset, and the crash he foresees could be the impetus for a chaotic reset, if one isn't proactively implemented before the crash occurs.

In "Aftermath", his most recent book published before the current pandemic (Kindle edition published October 2018)[128], he says:

> On form, the world is overdue for a new international monetary conference to implement a true global monetary reset. The most pressing question for monetary elites is whether a conference is convened proactively with a view to creating a coherent system, or convened reactively in the midst of a new global financial crisis likely to produce a draconian response. A crucial moment in monetary history has arrived.

Obviously that conference didn't happen before the pandemic hit, unless it did so behind closed doors and wasn't reported.

Is this pandemic that "crucial moment in monetary history", facilitating draconian restrictions on freedom of movement, while allowing central

---

[128] https://www.amazon.com/Aftermath-Secrets-Wealth-Preservation-Coming-ebook/dp/B07CV4SX82/

banks around the world to begin the process of implementing new digital currency systems?

Or are we in the final days of the current financial system, the calm before the storm, unaware of the financial chaos to come?

If we're heading swiftly into a world of digital currencies, then theoretically a crash could be avoided, or at least pushed further into the future, as unlimited currency could be created and distributed with just a few strokes on a keyboard. The dangers of a run on the banks, when everybody wants their cash out at the same time would also be negated, as all savings would be held digitally, with cash becoming a forgotten relic.

Once all transactions are conducted digitally, and cash is no longer used, every purchase you make can be tracked, analysed and controlled.

We're already heading in that direction. This "war on cash" has been on-going for several years. This EU (European Union) initiative[129] discusses the purported reasons:

> Cash has the important feature of offering anonymity to transactions. Such anonymity can be misused. The possibility to conduct large cash payments in particular facilitates money laundering and terrorist financing activities because of the difficulty to control cash payment transactions.

Since September 2015 France no longer allows its citizens to conduct any transaction above €1,000 in cash. The reasons, as stated by the French Government in 2015[130]:

> The circulation of large amounts of cash, and more generally the means of making anonymous payments, limits the traceability of these payments and the ability to fight against the financing of terrorism. Finance Minister Michel Sapin said to Reuters that the measure is 'necessary to fight against the use of cash and anonymity in the French economy'.

It is suggested that the real reason behind this push for a cashless society is more about tracking all transactions to facilitate more efficient tax collection and less about terrorism.

---

[129] https://ec.europa.eu/info/consultations/eu-initiative-restrictions-payments-cash_en

[130] https://www.frenchentree.com/blog/cash-payments-in-france-restricted-to-e1000/

Governments the world over are keen to insert themselves into every transaction between private individuals and take "their share" in the form of one tax or another. Digital currencies, coupled with larger cash transactions being made illegal makes this reality a done deal.

And the pandemic has hastened the move towards this digitalization.

On the other hand, if there is no proactive move to a more resilient system of control of all our finances, then perhaps we're in the final stages of a redistribution of the wealth before the system collapses.

Again, from James Rickard's "Aftermath":

> A struggling middle class has more to do with the future than the present. While today's numbers testify to the presence of a large middle class, their mood is pessimistic. There is a feeling that children will not do as well as their parents. There is a feeling of job insecurity. There is a feeling of overtaxation relative to other echelons of society. Above all, there is a feeling of a rigged game in which the rich share inside information, the poor are subsidized, and the middle class does all the work and receives no respect from elites or political leadership. None of these feelings is misplaced. Burdens placed on the middle class have never been greater, even as society's rewards are snatched by super-rich investors or recipients of government assistance.

This was published in late 2018. Have things improved for the burdened middle class since the pandemic began? Several studies show that the super-rich have become even richer, thanks to direct and indirect help from their governmental buddies. A quick search for the term "pandemic rich become richer" produces these articles as the top 5 search results:

- NBC News[131]: World's richest become wealthier during Covid pandemic as inequality grows
- MSN[132]: These 47 Billionaires Got Richer During the Pandemic
- NPR[133]: How The Pandemic Made The Ultra-Rich Even Richer

---

131 https://www.nbcnews.com/news/world/world-s-richest-become-wealthier-during-covid-pandemic-inequality-grows-n1255506

132 https://www.msn.com/en-us/money/savingandinvesting/these-47-billionaires-got-richer-during-the-pandemic/ss-BB19X4Zm

133 https://www.npr.org/2020/12/23/949606432/how-the-pandemic-made-the-ultra-rich-even-richer?t=1613390424036

- Forbes[134]: The Rich Are Getting Richer During The Pandemic
- CBS News[135]: U.S. billionaires gained almost $1 trillion in wealth during the pandemic

Follow the money. Who has benefitted the most from this crisis?

In his new book, entitled "The New Great Depression"[136], written after the pandemic began, and published on 12th January 2021, Rickards suggests that the lockdowns in reaction to the viral outbreak are going to result in economic misery the likes of which this generation has never seen:

> Depressions are more than statistics. A depression is the incalculable sum of individual traumas from job losses and concerns about paying the rent, putting food on the table, securing health care, and helping children get a good education. Job losses do not affect only paychecks; they affect dignity, self-confidence, and prospects for the future. And depressions are more than job losses. Businesses are destroyed or at best disrupted. Ripples extend from there to communities and entire cities. The impact of a depression is deep and long lasting; it may be intergenerational, as was the case with the first Great Depression.

Follow the money. Who stands to lose the most when the appalling economic consequences of lockdowns and business closures eventually play out in full?

What conclusions do you arrive at when following the money?

---

134 https://www.forbes.com/sites/jackkelly/2020/07/22/the-rich-are-getting-richer-during-the-pandemic/

135 https://www.cbsnews.com/news/billionaires-pandemic-1-trillion-wealth-gain/

136 https://www.amazon.com/New-Great-Depression-Winners-Post-Pandemic-ebook/dp/B08DMVQ184/

PART 7:
THE DECISIONS WE MAKE

"I'll tell you what they [the global elite] don't want. They don't want a population of citizens capable of critical thinking. They don't want well informed, well educated people capable of critical thinking. They're not interested in that. That doesn't help them."

George Carlin

Critical thinking

The quote used to introduce this final section is from George Carlin[137], stand-up comedian, actor, social critic and author. I'd like to include the quote in full here, because it is key to understanding why all of this matters, and why it is so important to develop your critical thinking abilities:

> "Because the owners of this country don't want that. I'm talking about the real owners now, the big wealthy business interests that control things and make all the important decisions. Forget the politicians, they're irrelevant. The politicians are put there to give you the idea you have freedom of choice. You don't. You have no choice. You have owners. They own you. They own everything. They own all the important land, they own and control the corporations that've long since bought and paid for, the senate, the congress, the state houses, the city halls, they got the judges in their back pocket, and they own all the big media companies so they control just about all of the news and the information you get to hear. They got you by the balls. They spend billions of dollars every year lobbying to get what they want. Well, we know what they want. They want more for themselves and less for everybody else. But I'll tell you what they don't want. They don't want a population of citizens capable of critical thinking. They don't want well informed, well educated people capable of critical thinking. They're not interested in that. That doesn't help them."
>
> George Carlin

You can watch George's rant on stage in New York in a short YouTube clip entitled "You Have Owners":
https://www.youtube.com/watch?v=H-PSCqhkWhg

So what exactly is critical thinking, and how do we develop our ability to develop our skills?

The Foundation For Critical Thinking[138] provides the following definition:

> Critical thinking is the intellectually disciplined process of actively and skillfully conceptualizing, applying, analyzing, synthesizing, and/or evaluating information gathered from, or generated by, observation, experience, reflection, reasoning, or communication, as a guide to belief and action.

---

[137] https://en.wikipedia.org/wiki/George_Carlin

[138] https://www.criticalthinking.org/pages/defining-critical-thinking/766

The key part, in terms of the decision you're weighing up by reading this book, is "as a guide to belief and action". You have a choice to make, and the more clearly you consider all the information you can gather to assist you, the better, hopefully, you will be equipped to make the right decision for your own personal circumstances.

The Foundation For Critical Thinking continue, by suggesting critical thinking can be seen as having two components:

1) a set of information and belief generating and processing skills
2) the habit, based on intellectual commitment, of using those skills to guide behavior.

The University of Louisville breaks down the meaning of critical thinking into a few useful bulletpoint descriptions[139]:

> Critical thinking has been described as an ability to
>
> - question
> - acknowledge and test previously held assumptions
> - recognize ambiguity
> - examine, interpret, evaluate, reason, and reflect
> - make informed judgments and decisions

This also provides a useful framework for what we're trying to achieve here. We are certainly questioning, and there is no doubt that there is plenty of ambiguity in the information that is presented to us. But through careful consideration we hope we will be better prepared to make an informed judgement and a rational decision.

Gathering information

One of the first steps is to gather information from as wide a range of sources as possible. This is actually harder than it should be, due to the on-going censorship efforts of Big Tech, the media, and those trying to control the pro-vaccine narrative.

"When truth is replaced by silence, the silence is a lie."

Yevgeny Yevtushenko

By avoiding the platforms and tools that seem to want to silence dissenting voices, or push your attention in a particular direction, you have a better chance of gathering useful information.

---

139 https://louisville.edu/ideastoaction/about/criticalthinking/what

So instead of using Google Chrome as your browser you might want to look at changing to Brave browser. You'll find the experience very similar, but there is no tracking of your activity in order to feed you adverts the tech giant wants you to see. In fact many adverts are blocked, so you tend to get a cleaner, faster browsing experience.

Next, stop using Google Search. Instead try using Duck Duck Go, which doesn't feed different search results to different people, or track your previous searches and activity. You'll probably find you get a more balanced set of options for any term you search for.

If you're looking for videos on certain topics, don't just stick to YouTube, where many alternative viewpoints are censored and deleted. There are other video websites where videos featuring content which runs against the main narrative are never removed. Here are a couple of places those who have been "cancelled" by Google (who own YouTube) have found a more open-minded reception:

LBRY: https://lbry.tv/

Odysee: https://odysee.com/

BitChute: https://www.bitchute.com/

Rumble: https://rumble.com/

Banned Video: https://banned.video/

Brand New Tube: https://brandnewtube.com/

Read alternative websites with an open mind, rather than listening to those who would quickly discount these sites and their authors as crackpot conspiracy theorists.

If you use social media sites, be aware that your Facebook and Twitter feeds are collated to fit the AI algorithm's assessment of your interests and biases. What you are seeing is not a representation of all information and viewpoints available.

You'll find some interesting ideas and links in the comments of videos, even on YouTube. You'll be able to gauge the level of agreement or disagreement on issues you're researching, as people usually feel they can express themselves freely and honestly if they are anonymous or semi-anonymous online. You'll also find links to other videos, articles, news stories, and more.

Follow your instincts and interests, and see where these links take you. You never know what you'll find, and how that might impact your own thinking process.

Assessing information

Question everything.

Don't assume that any article you read, or any video you watch is telling you the truth. Remember, as we discussed earlier, all most people are offering is an opinion, more often than not based upon the opinions of other sources they have studied.

Anyone who passionately presents their opinion as "the truth" should be subject to even further scrutiny. Why are they so fiercely attached to their own particular viewpoint? They are much less likely to be open-minded and impartial in what they present than someone who freely admits they don't have the "facts", but simply has thoughts and ideas based upon rational thinking.

> "The opinions that are held with passion are always those for which no good ground exists; indeed the passion is the measure of the holder's lack of rational conviction. Opinions in politics ... are almost always held passionately."
>
> Bertrand Russell

Consider the sources when accessing information from mainstream media. What are their beliefs, what is their motivation? Are they independent, or beholden to an editor who may have a different agenda? Is there a parent company which may have undue influence over the content of articles published?

Making a decision

Arriving at a conclusion isn't something that has to happen at a certain pre-selected moment in time, in the traditional "It's decision time!" model. You'll find that your thoughts and ideas evolve over time as you consider more information from more sources.

Don't be afraid to adjust your position in the light of new information, or when presented with new ideas. Your decision doesn't need to be set in stone and defended at all costs. If you find your opinion shifting that is just a part of the process.

But remember, in this current dilemma a decision must be made at some point. And if you don't decide for yourself, you are allowing others to make the decision for you.

> "Courage doesn't happen when you have all the answers. It happens when you are ready to face the questions you have been avoiding..."
>
> Shannon L. Alder

Censorship

Here are a few quotes on the topic of censorship, the first two coming from previous presidents of the United States. Truman was 33rd president, from 1945 to 1953:

> "Once a government is committed to the principle of silencing the voice of opposition, it has only one way to go, and that is down the path of increasingly repressive measures, until it becomes a source of terror to all its citizens and creates a country where everyone lives in fear."
>
> Harry S. Truman

Truman was succeded by Eisenhower who held power from 1953 to 1961:

> "Don't join the book burners. Don't think you're going to conceal faults by concealing evidence that they ever existed. Don't be afraid to go in your library and read every book..."
>
> Dwight D. Eisenhower

Censorship is insulting to us as adults, capable of thinking for ourselves, considering what is going on around us, and responsible for making our own choices about our own life. What gives one group of people the right to tell another what they can or can't see, listen to or read?

> "Censorship is telling a man he can't have a steak just because a baby can't chew it."
>
> Mark Twain

One has to question the motives when someone decides to censor a particular video, article or book. Why do they want to silence certain ideas, or brand those who put forward alternative possibilities as conspiracy theorists?

> "When you tear out a man's tongue, you are not proving him a liar, you're only telling the world that you fear what he might say."
>
> George R.R. Martin

The easiest conclusion to draw when material which questions a particular narrative is censored is that those doing the censoring really do fear the message, most likely because someone is getting too close to the truth.

I'll let the United Nations have the last word on the matter of censorship in their Universal Declaration of Human Rights:

> "Everyone has the right to freedom of opinion and expression; this right includes freedom to hold opinions without interference and to seek, receive and impart information and ideas through any media and regardless of frontiers."
>
> United Nations
>
> Universal Declaration of Human Rights

Subtle manipulation

We'll finish this section with a look at how language can be used as a subtle form of persuasion, even manipulation. If you don't question everything as you research and gather your thoughts, it is easy to be subconsciously swayed by what amounts to subtle propaganda.

Let's begin by reading this 18th January 2021 article from NBC News[140], which is very positively biased towards the "everybody must be vaccinated" narrative:

ARTICLE: Covid misinformation takes its toll on British doctors, teachers

The title itself is subtly suggesting that all that will be discussed in the article is misinformation, and that this heavy burden of lies is "taking its toll" on our heroic doctors.

> British front-line workers who were applauded on doorsteps in the early weeks of the pandemic now confront a torrent of polarization and misinformation.

"A torrent of polarization and misinformation". That's a pretty strong introduction. A torrent would suggest an overwhelming, unstoppable flood.

> Doctors, teachers and other exhausted workers say they are feeling incredibly demoralized after reading social media posts insisting Covid-19 is a hoax or overblown. And that has had serious, real-world consequences in recent weeks, with demonstrators picketing hospitals and hurling abuse at health care staff.

If you're "demoralized" by reading social media posts, I suggest you stay off social media for a while. Everybody is entitled to an opinion, and is entitled to express that opinion. Refer back to the United Nations' Universal Declaration of Human Rights (previous section) if in doubt about this. Just because someone believes that "Covid-19 is overblown" doesn't mean they are spreading misinformation. They are merely expressing an opinion.

> Some researchers say the polarization between British people who are sucked in by these ideas and those who aren't is becoming more extreme — and in turn more like the United States.

---

[140] https://www.nbcnews.com/news/world/covid-misinformation-takes-its-toll-british-doctors-teachers-n1254568

"Sucked in by these ideas"! Yes, anybody who believes such nonsense must be an absolute idiot. Obviously the government- and pharma-spun tales make so much more sense.

> This spiraling "infodemic" — as the World Health Organization calls it — comes as the United Kingdom deals with a surge in coronavirus cases, forcing the country to enter its third national lockdown and pushing its beloved, publicly funded National Health Service close to the breaking point.

The "infodemic" that is "spiraling" has little, if any, link to the surge in cases, but the article, without directly saying so, links these two ideas in the same paragraph – in fact in the same sentence. Are they suggesting the "infodemic" pushing our "beloved, publicly funded" (for 'publicly funded', read 'taxpayer funded') health service to the brink.

Conspiracy theories are far from new here, and Britain has grappled with coronavirus-related misinformation since the start of the pandemic.

Ah, there we are, "conspiracy theories". The default "de-bunk those with questions" fallback position. Don't worry, these idiots who think that "Covid-19 is overblown" are just voicing their deluded conspiracy theories. Nothing to see here.

The article continues under a sub-heading in quotes: "Covid is a hoax".

Read on yourself, and look for further bias, and subtle (or not so subtle) use of language in an attempt to manipulate your opinion of anyone who dares to question the narrative.

Here are just a couple of my favourite choice phrases from the remainder of the article:

- peddling fake news
- crazy conspiracy theories
- Britain is buckling under
- anti-vaxxers and Covid-deniers
- right-wing news sites
- a very dangerous message

In conclusion, try to practice reading more consciously, and ask what the writer is trying to say in his article. What is his agenda? What does he believe?

And what does he want you to believe?

CONCLUSIONS

"Who you are tomorrow begins with what you do today."

Tim Fargo

Vaccine roundup

Let's revisit briefly the opening statements of this book.

I made the point that I don't have any answers for you.

Therefore I feel the need to apologise once again, because a lack of any definitive answers, or even any concrete conclusions, means that you will have to make your own decisions, based on your own assessment of what you see happening around you.

I can't be sure about what is actually going on. I think it is almost impossible for anyone to make such a claim in today's world of 24-hour "news", endless political spin, hidden financial incentives and overt censorship.

The claims made by anyone who presents their information as "the facts" must be viewed with a healthy dose of scepticism. What they are really presenting is their opinion, based on the evidence they have available to them. This evidence comes from other sources who are also often expressing their own opinions, basing what they say on yet more opinions from other sources.

The line between "facts" and "opinion" is very blurred. Obviously the closer a person is to discussing matters in their own personal field of expertise, the more likely they are to be correct in the conclusions they draw, and the information they present. Although even then, one must throw some consideration of motives into the mix.

As an example, a well-established vaccine company can reasonably be considered to be expert in their field. But when they rush out an experimental treatment, authorised for use under emergency guidelines only, and yet claim it is both safe and effective, one must consider the potential billions of dollars of profit a worldwide roll-out will create.

The truth, then, must lie somewhere between the two extremes of current possibility:

1) That everything we are told in the media, and by our politicians, medical agencies and big pharma companies is completely true: the virus is spreading out of control, it is deadly, there is no credible treatment, there is an urgent need for mass vaccination, and the vaccines are safe and effective.
2) That a pandemic, either genuine or manufactured, is being used as a smokescreen for various nefarious ends by a shady world elite, who wish to grab more power, money, security and control over the population of the world.

I really still don't know where my opinion falls on this spectrum ranging from benign mitigation to evil dictatorship. But, in my opinion, there are just far too many inconsistencies in the stories we are told to simply accept the narrative we are all being fed.

My most hopeful conclusion is that this is all simply about big pharma mega-profits, and that their financial influence in government policy and media outlets is what is helping drive the push for hurried vaccination for all.

However, if it is just about the money, that doesn't excuse them using us all as experimental sheep to be regularly rounded up and shorn for profit.

There are many darker conclusions that can be drawn, and you don't have to dig too deep, or think too hard, to imagine more ominous ultimate outcomes. Sheep are rounded up to be shorn regularly until their usefulness as wool producers expires. Once they become a burden rather than an asset, they are rounded up for a final time to be processed as mutton.

So, if I can't provide answers the best I can offer is the opportunity for you to give some considered thought to the "unprecedented" situation we find ourselves in.

At times like this it would be so easy to simply give in to peer pressure, and the optimistic hope that when everyone has been vaccinated, everything will return to some sort of pre-COVID normality.

In fact this would probably be the prudent choice to make, because in the current hysterical climate, anyone who so much as dares to question the vaccine narrative is branded a "cov-idiot", a "vaccine denier", a "conspiracy theorist", or in some extreme circumstances, a "selfish murderer" !

But if you've got this far in the book I'm assuming you're not one to simply follow the herd, at least not without putting some thought into your decision first.

So, having outlined many of the topics you might like to think about, ponder, discuss and consider, I'll try to boil down the decision making process to one simple question...

Do you believe the narrative?

Do you wholly believe the narrative behind the push to vaccinate the entire world?

To help you answer this, here are a few of the topics we have raised for consideration:

- Are we being told the truth, the whole truth, and nothing but the truth?
- Do you feel you can put your full trust in all the players involved and invested in getting that needle into your arm?
- Do you think there is a global elite pulling the strings of power from high above, and if so, do they have your best interests at heart?
- Can you trust your government, and are they doing the best job they can of managing a real crisis?
- Do you trust the pharma giants who have produced novel, experimental vaccines in world-record-breaking timeframes, who have asserted (based on results from their own trials) that the vaccines are safe and effective, and have then rushed those vaccines through Emergency Use Authorizations?
- Do you believe Big Pharma's main priority is the health and wellbeing of the world's population?
- Do you believe the vaccine is both safe and effective, and will help the world return to normal?
- Are you happy to (probably) receive a fresh vaccine each year, like an annual flu shot?
- Do you trust the media narrative around this enthusiastic headlong dash into medically uncertain waters?
- Do you believe the media, which is mostly controlled by a few huge international conglomerates, is still entirely impartial and truthful, without any other agenda?
- Do you trust the opinions of others in your society who are prepared to berate you for merely daring to question what is going on?

If you can answer a big resounding "YES" to this key question, and you're confident that everyone involved in the headlong rush into vaccination is acting purely out of concern for the population of the world, then your decision is a simple one.

If you have any doubts about what is happening, and feel that something just doesn't seem right about the narrative constantly being pushed forward, then you have a bit more thinking to do, and a personal decision to make.

Are you ready to be a part of the "The Great Vaccine Roundup of 2021", or are you going to step aside for a while and see how things develop?

If we truly live in the free society we're constantly told we enjoy, then the choice is yours and yours alone to make, and you should feel no pressure from any quarter once you've made your decision.

Whatever you decide, I wish you a healthy and prosperous future.

Let us know what you think at:
https://VaccineRoundup.com

What next?

If you have decided against vaccination, what do you do next?

Well, that really depends on where you think all this is going. If you think the best case, least malignant scenario is in play – that this is just about big pharma mega-profits – then you can potentially sidestep any risks by refusing a vaccine, and hope all returns to normal when the Big Vaccine Roundup is complete.

But if you're worried we're heading for vaccine mandates, vaccine passports, more lockdowns, virus mutations and ever-on-going vaccine booster shots, or other restrictions on our movements and freedom, then things aren't going to get any better if you just do nothing.

My own personal conclusion is that there is a lot more going on in this story than we see at the moment. That is why I felt it necessary to write this book. There are lots of books that present the wildest, darkest theories as "the truth". Maybe they're right, but for the average person on the street these ideas are just a bit "too far out there".

I wanted to write something a bit more balanced, something that simply encourages people to at least ask a few questions, something that people might feel comfortable sharing with their friends and family.

Other than potential income from book sales, I don't really have anything to gain by sticking my neck out like this. In fact, it is quite likely I'll get myself branded as a "conspiracy theorist", or even an "extremist"[141]. But I

---

141 https://www.independent.co.uk/news/uk/home-news/coronavirus-social-media-anti-vax-misinformation-vaccine-conspiracy-a9604481.html

From the July 2020 article on TheIndependent.co.uk website:

> "If 31 per cent of people do not take the vaccine we will not achieve herd immunity," Imran Ahmed, chief executive of the CCDH (The Centre for Countering Digital Hate), told The Independent.
>
> "If we don't reach that we will not be able to contain the virus. We will have waves and waves of years and years and tens of thousands of people will die."

Later in the article Imran Ahmen also says:

> "But I would go beyond calling anti-vaxxers conspiracy theorists to say they are an extremist group that pose a national security risk."

Mr. Ahmed's organization has published a 54 page PDF file called "The Anti-Vaxx Playbook". You can find it here: (continued at foot of next page...)

couldn't just sit back and say nothing and maintain a clear conscience. I felt I needed to share my thoughts.

If you feel this way too, then I'd be very grateful if you would consider doing a couple of things:

- If you found value in this book, please consider writing a review on Amazon. It really does help.
- Also please consider sharing the book with your loved ones in any way you feel comfortable doing so.

We need to share information outside of the control of those who would wish to censor anything that goes against their narrative. How do we do this? The best way is to share in the old fashioned way, person to person, by word-of-mouth recommendation.

If you are concerned about what is going on, and about the effort to silence those who simply want to ask questions, then by sharing your thoughts with your loved ones you are helping to put more people in a position of strength, able to do their own critical thinking, and make their own informed decisions.

If most of the population ask no questions, and simply go along with the "all must be vaccinated" narrative, then as we reach ever greater percentages of the population who have been vaccinated, it isn't hard to imagine that those wielding authority will see this as implied approval to mandate that the stragglers to be rounded up and inoculated against their will, as they are selfishly "endangering lives".

Even if this eventual outcome doesn't come via government mandate, it is easy to see how encouraging private businesses to require a vaccine certificate before someone can access their services will force most people to comply anyway. Want to go take a flight? Already, according to Qantas in Australia[142], you'll need your "vaccine passport". Once restaurants, bars, gyms, cinemas and supermarkets follow like sheep, vaccination will be necessary just to take part in day-to-day life.

Do nothing, and it's possible you'll find yourself on the pointed end of a needle regardless of your preferences. If you care about remaining a free,

---

https://www.counterhate.com/playbook

It's only a small step from being labelled an "extremist" who poses a threat to national security to being categorized as a domestic terrorist.

[142] https://www.abc.net.au/news/2020-11-24/covid-19-vaccine-passport-australia-qantas/12914246

sovereign individual, with the right to decide what gets put into your body and what doesn't, then please share.

If we all just sit back and do nothing, then we all lose, as those with a hidden agenda will be able to push it through with minimal resistance. When that leads to more loss of freedoms, more vaccine mandates, and more economic misery, then we'll have nobody to blame but ourselves.

Thank you.

Ian Usher

February 2021

APPENDIX A: RESOURCES

In writing this book I've tried wherever possible to use reliable and trusted sources, and have included footnotes in the text whenever I have quoted something directly. However, as stated multiple times throughout the book, the veracity of anything quoted is hard to measure, so all links are offered merely for you to form your own opinions, not as any assertion of "fact".

Here are some of the sources I found to be particularly useful while compiling this book. This isn't intended to be an exhaustive list of all the resources I referred to, but is a good starting point for your own research.

Watch, read, listen, question, and follow your own instincts in order to reach your own conclusions.

Documentaries

Silence On Vaccine (aka "Shots In The Dark") (2009)

https://www.imdb.com/title/tt2172632/

Silent Epidemic: The Untold Story of Vaccines (2013)

https://www.imdb.com/title/tt3290196/

Trace Amounts (2014)

https://www.imdb.com/title/tt3715598/

Vaxxed: From Cover-Up to Catastrophe (2016)

https://www.imdb.com/title/tt5562652/

https://vaxxedthemovie.com/

Vaxxed 2 - The Peoples Truth (2019)

https://www.imdb.com/title/tt11137248/

https://www.vaxxed2.com/

1986: The Act (2020)

https://www.imdb.com/title/tt12708236/

The Social Dilemma (2020)

https://www.imdb.com/title/tt11464826/

https://www.netflix.com/title/81254224

Plandemic 1: The Hidden Agenda Behind COVID-19 (2020)

https://www.imdb.com/title/tt12927010/

This video can be freely accessed at the BitChute "officialplandemic" channel here:

https://www.bitchute.com/video/JtPTJmnlWDq0/

Plandemic 2: Indoctornation (2020)

https://www.imdb.com/title/tt12927074/

This video can be freely accessed at the BitChute "officialplandemic" channel here:

https://www.bitchute.com/video/4u7rt61YeGox/

This video now has over 1 million views on BitChute alone, and is very good as a "follow the money" deep dive. Highly recommended.

Books

"The man who does not read has no advantage over the man who cannot read."

Mark Twain

Unreported Truths About Covid-19 and Lockdowns: Combined Parts 1-3: Death Counts, Lockdowns, and Masks

by Alex Berenson

https://www.amazon.com/Unreported-Truths-About-Covid-19-Lockdowns-ebook/dp/B08QND25GL/

NOTE: Don't make the mistake of buying similarly titled books by "Allan Barenston" or "Andrew Brinston", which aren't (in my opinion) anywhere near as good as this (originally banned) book.

Vaccines Are Dangerous - And Don't Work

Dr Vernon Coleman

https://www.amazon.com/Vaccines-Are-Dangerous-Dont-Work-ebook/dp/B00HSSRK1E/

Lots of information from a doctor who has much experience in this field.

I Do Not Consent: My Fight Against Medical Cancel Culture

Simone Gold MD JD

https://www.amazon.com/Do-Not-Consent-Against-Medical-ebook/dp/B08L8JK7FL/

A fascinating overview of one doctor's amazement and disbelief at the lengths authorities have gone to discredit doctors who believe HCQ can be used as a very effective treatment.

Scamdemic - The COVID-19 Agenda: The Liberal's Plot To Win The White House

by John Iovine

https://www.amazon.com/Scamdemic-COVID-19-Agenda-Liberals-White-ebook/dp/B08DHMYQNK/

Has some interesting points, but has heavy political bias too.

Aftermath: Seven Secrets of Wealth Preservation in the Coming Chaos

by James Rickards

https://www.amazon.com/Aftermath-Secrets-Wealth-Preservation-Coming-ebook/dp/B07CV4SX82/

In-depth look at the global economy, and troubles that may lie ahead.

The New Great Depression: Winners and Losers in a Post-Pandemic World

by James Rickards

https://www.amazon.com/New-Great-Depression-Winners-Post-Pandemic-ebook/dp/B08DMVQ184/

Follow-up to "Aftermath", written after the start of the pandemic, looking at potential financial consequences.

Websites

https://www.americasfrontlinedocs.com/

https://c19study.com/

https://c19ivermectin.com/

https://covid19criticalcare.com/

https://goldsilver.com/

https://healthimpactnews.com/

https://www.historyofvaccines.org/

https://thelightpaper.co.uk/

https://medicalkidnap.com/

https://www.mercola.com/

https://off-guardian.org/

https://www.peakprosperity.com/

https://projects.propublica.org/docdollars/

https://stevenguinness2.wordpress.com/

https://www.theatlantic.com/

https://thevaccinereaction.org/

https://vaccineimpact.com/

https://vaccinedeaths.com/

https://www.vernoncoleman.com/

https://www.weforum.org/

https://www.zerohedge.com/

"Adverse event reports" (death)

This link should give you immediate access to the most recent count of deaths reported to VAERS (Vaccine Adverse Event Reporting System) after taking a vaccine, split into age categories.

https://medalerts.org/vaersdb/findfield.php?TABLE=ON&GROUP1=AGE&EVENTS=ON&ESORT=VAX-DATE&VAX=COVID19&DIED=Yes

APPENDIX B: ACRONYMS

Delving into the world of government departments and policies involves entering a veritable alphabet soup of acronyms. Here are the most common ones referred to in the book:

BMJ	British Medical Journal
CBRN	Chemical, Biological, Radiological and Nuclear
CDC	Centers for Disease Control and Prevention
CPNI	Centre for the Protection of the National Infrastructure
DG	Director-General
DHSC	Department of Health and Social Care
ECB	European Central Bank
EU	European Union
EUA	Emergency Use Authorization
FDA	Food and Drug Administration
ICL	Imperial College London
ICU	Intensive Care Unit
IMF	International Monetary Fund
NCVIA	The National Childhood Vaccine Injury Act (1986)
NERVTAG	New and Emerging Respiratory Virus Threats Advisory Group
NHS	National Health Service
NIAID	The National Institute of Allergy and Infectious Diseases
NIH	National Institutes of Health
NVICP	National Vaccine Injury Compensation Program
OPEC	Organization of the Petroleum Exporting Countries
PCR Test	Polymerase Chain Reaction Test
PHE	Public Health England
PHEIC	Public Health Emergency of International Concern
PPE	Personal Protective Equipment
PREP Act	Public Readiness and Emergency Preparedness Act
RT-PCR	Reverse Transcription Polymerase Chain Reaction
SAGE	Scientific Advisory Group for Emergencies
UN	United Nations
VAERS	Vaccine Adverse Event Reporting System
WEF	World Economic Forum
WHO	World Health Organization
WIV	Wuhan Institute of Virology

ABOUT THE AUTHOR

Find out more about the author in his two previous autobiographical books:

A LIFE SOLD: What ever happened to that guy who sold his whole life on eBay? (2010)

https://www.amazon.com/LIFE-SOLD-What-happened-whole-ebook/dp/B004FN1V1A/

What on earth would make someone decide to put their whole life up for sale… on eBay?

When Ian Usher decided that it was time to leave the past behind and move on to the next chapter of his life, that is exactly what he did. The results were surprising, entertaining and challenging.

However, the auction was only the beginning of the adventure. What does someone do when they have sold their life? Well, just about anything they like really!

Armed with a list of 100 lifetime goals, and a self-imposed timeframe of 100 weeks, Ian embarked on what could truly be described as the journey of a lifetime – a global adventure spanning six continents, two years, and almost every emotion.

From the amazing highs of achievement, happiness and love, to the terrible lows of disappointment, loneliness and despair, come along and enjoy the rollercoaster ride of life, as experienced by one traveller who is simply looking for a new start.

Paradise Delayed: Our new lives in the wild. Caribbean island life in the beautiful archipelago of Bocas del Toro, Panama (2014)

https://www.amazon.com/Paradise-Delayed-Caribbean-beautiful-archipelago-ebook/dp/B00C5PDTOM/

What does someone do after putting their whole life up for sale on eBay, then travelling the world for two years with a list of 100 lifetime goals and a challenging timeframe of 100 weeks, and finally selling the rights for the whole amazing story to Walt Disney Pictures?

Why, they go and buy their own private Caribbean island, of course!

The author's continuing quest for amazing adventures and incredible experiences take him to the beautiful tropical archipelago of Bocas del Toro, on the Caribbean coast of Panama. There he somehow ends up purchasing his own private Caribbean island - it sounds like a dream come true, doesn't it?

Maybe not! The trials and tribulations of a gringo trying to make a home on an overgrown island make for a fascinating portrayal of life in this challenging area of the world.

Sinking boats, defective chainsaws, document forgery and aggressive roosters are just a small sample of the hurdles facing a tired traveller who really just wants to lie in a hammock sipping margaritas for a while!

"Paradise Delayed" may make you re-consider the nature of the Caribbean island dream, or may just inspire to find your own adventure of a lifetime.

This newly updated version of "Paradise ...delayed" contains 16 new chapters chronicling more tropical adventures and mishaps, including details of the filming of a documentary TV show at the island, appropriately titled "New Lives in the Wild".

Website

https://IanUsher.com

www.ingramcontent.com/pod-product-compliance
Ingram Content Group UK Ltd.
Pitfield, Milton Keynes, MK11 3LW, UK
UKHW042018190726
13854UKWH00005B/2343